The Art and Practice of Dance/Movement Therapy

Linda S. Behar-Horenstein
University of Florida
Jane Ganet-Sigel
Columbia College

Please visit our website at www.pearsoncustom.com

ISBN 0–536–02420–0

BA 990144

PEARSON CUSTOM PUBLISHING
160 Gould Street/Needham Heights, MA 02494
A Pearson Education Company

Table of Contents

List of Tables and Figures

Acknowledgements

The development of this book has been a long process. Many people were involved in the data collection, research, support, and encouragement of this project. Without their gracious assistance and diligent work, completing this text would have become infinitely more challenging. We would like to thank the following individuals: Sandra Anusavice for her diligence in the meticulous transcription of interview tapes, procurement of research articles, careful editing of multiple drafts of the work and her continuous interest, dedication, curiosity, and enthusiasm; Andrea Brown, for her wisdom and the many lessons that I have learned from her over the many years of our friendship, her belief in the project, and the copious editorial assistance she offered, Rita Sutker, and the many individuals who were willing to be interviewed even though in many cases, they had never met Linda. The interviewees' passion and support for this project was incalculable and a catalyst in its own right that provided momentum to moving this work towards completion. We want to acknowledge Hal Hawkins, our editor at Pearson Publishing Solutions, for his support, encouragement, and enthusiasm for this project. Many thanks for taking on the publication of this novel topic. Also a debt of gratitude is owed to Terry Gets, our representative from Allyn & Bacon who affirmed our belief that this publication was indeed important and timely, and urged us to contact Hal Hawkins.

I owe an enormous debt of gratitude to my family. To my husband, Ben, whose enduring faith, love, and belief in the need for this book soothed me when the time crunch of juggling the roles of mother, wife, and professor were operating in conflict with the fact that there really are only 24 hours in any given day. To my children, Rachel and Max. Rachel was about 9 months when I began writing. As this project grew, it also was witness to the creation of new life, and Rachel was joined by her baby brother, Max. Their innate curiosity, spiritedness, exuberance and love for life has been a source of joy. Ben, Rachel, and Max have indeed made me feel like a very lucky woman.

During the development of this text, Jane suffered a serious stroke. She lost the ability to speak and write, but that didn't stop her. After regaining these capacities, despite immeasurable mitigating factors, she re-assumed her role as the Chair of the Graduate Program of Dance/Movement Therapy at Columbia College in Chicago. About six months before this book went to press, she decided that she wanted more time to consult and enjoy her family, so at the tender age of 73 she retired. In recognition of her contributions to the field and Columbia College, the administration honored her with emeritus status.

Linda Behar-Horenstein dedicates this book to her mother, for giving her the gifts to endure a journey into darkness, to Jane for patiently and persistently guiding her back into the light, and to her husband Ben for his friendship, love, and constancy.

Jane Ganet-Sigel dedicates this book to her parents, Goldye and Leonard Mendelssohn, for their undying support and sensitivity, to her children, Marcey, Fred, Larry, and Edward, for flowing beautifully through many changes, and to her husband Mel, who has lovingly danced through life with her.

Foreword

Andrea K. Brown
Linda S. Behar-Horenstein

That which cannot be spoken, can be sung
That which cannot be sung, can be danced
— French saying

On the journey called life, if you are lucky, you will meet a very special person who unlocks life's treasures. For us, that very special person is Jane Ganet-Sigel. The key she gave us is dance/movement therapy. Life's journey can feel painful and wounding because needs are not optimally met. Unfortunately, because no human environment is perfect, some needs are inevitably not taken care of. This is part of the human condition. Life's treasures can be overshadowed by pains and wounds. Dance/movement therapy can be a means for healing those wounds and addressing unmet needs.

As a witness to Jane's work as a teacher, therapist, mentor, and colleague, we have seen her bring vitality to the lives of others in so many ways. We are especially pleased that this book presents Jane Ganet-Sigel's approach to the principles of dance/movement therapy in a way that can enable more people to understand and appreciate them. Jane helps those who have contact with her to gain a fuller sense of self.

Dance/movement therapy is a relatively young field when compared to science, mathematics, and humanities. The work of its founder, Marian Chace, charter members, practitioners, and its national organization, the American Dance Therapy Association has helped to shape its identity. In our quest to contribute to the writings about the history of the field and acknowledge the work of Jane Ganet-Sigel, we have tried to answer the following questions:

1. How can we advance an understanding and appreciation for the field of dance/movement therapy?

2. Who might benefit from learning about this therapeutic approach?

3. What can future dance/movement therapists learn from Jane Ganet Sigel's experiences in program development?

4. How can instruction help students make the transition from classroom experiences to becoming an effective therapist?

5. How has Jane Ganet-Sigel used instructional strategies to train therapists?

6. How do specific dance/movement therapy techniques influence the treatment of patients?

7. How has Jane Ganet-Sigel utilized dance/movement therapy techniques to facilitate patients' recovery?

The Art and Practice of Dance/Movement Therapy is written for therapists, educators, allied health professionals, dancers, and persons who are interested in exploring the vitality of alternative approaches to treating mental illness and the emotional components associated with physical illnesses. This book will serve scholars and students of dance/movement in the domains of teaching and learning and will support the training of practitioners. This textbook provides systematic approaches to developing curriculum and using instructional strategies, teaching for success, and illuminating how theoretical tenets can be applied in patient treatment.

The book is divided into three parts: The Theory and Practice of Dance/Movement Therapy, Cases in Dance/Movement Therapy, and A Comparison of Dance/Movement and Verbal Psychotherapies. Each part is preceded by a brief introduction. Each chapter begins with a set of guiding questions that are designed to focus the reader's attention on key concepts. Many books in the field have focused on an explication of theoretical frameworks, techniques, purposes, or case studies. In contrast the authors have explored issues related to theory, teaching, training, therapeutic practice, and research. They have tried to represent the depth and breadth of viewpoints in the field and have included discussion of issues that may be considered controversial.

The authors have tried to report the status of the field as portrayed by current research. They have also offered ideas about formulating research studies that may enhance understanding of just how potent dance/movement therapy may be in bringing about sustained healing. They have tried to contribute to the readers' understanding and appreciation of the historical developments within the field. Finally it is hoped that this book will preserve the legacy of Jane Ganet-Sigel whose work has helped to shape the field of dance/movement therapy and influence the thought and actions of others who work in allied fields.

Introduction

Many alternatives and adjuncts to traditional psychotherapy have emerged throughout the years, such as art therapy, music therapy, psychodrama, and dance/movement therapy. Each therapy offers a specific media and related techniques to help patients reveal feelings that they may have difficulty verbalizing. In dance/movement therapy, patients use body movement to access and reveal their innermost feelings. What is unique about dance/movement therapy is that it is the patients' feelings as expressed through movement, not the therapist, that provides the structure and influences the direction of therapy.

We live in a society that teaches us to be verbal and inadvertently being verbal becomes a way of distancing ourselves from our feelings and our bodies. Society also encourages some members to become silent and keep things inside. As a result people become quite adept at rationalization and compacting things in the body. Dance/movement therapy is an artful way to reawaken deadened parts of the body and psyche. Through the dance/movement therapy process individuals can become healthy.

Dance/movement therapy appeals to a diverse clientele. For example, it has been used for patients with eating disorders to facilitate their ability to identify feeling states, establish more realistic body perceptions, and heal their impoverished sense of self-esteem. For hospitalized patients, this form of therapy has helped individuals learn how to communicate in more acceptable ways, replace maladaptive movement, and develop alternative coping methods. Through dance/movement, geriatrics have regained feelings of self-worth and become revitalized. For children and adolescents with physical and mental disabilities, it offers a range of treatment by providing techniques specific to their personality or disability. For example, dance/movement therapy with children who are emotionally disturbed can provide a bridge from the child's tumultuous world to external reality and be used to help patients establish a trusting relationship with the dance therapist and later with others. Dance/movement therapy has been used in treatment for patients with substance abuse, Alzheimer's disease, and for those who are undergoing rehabilitation. Used also for outpatient treatment, it has enabled clients to lead more fulfilling lives by helping them gain adaptive coping mechanisms, replace dysfunctional messages and behaviors with satisfying ones, recognize changes in their viscera as a signal to move away from a painful situation, and change the way they use, inhibit, or abuse their bodies. Dance/movement has been recognized as a means to open the doors to treatment so tightly closed for many clients.

The American Dance/Movement Therapy Association defines dance movement therapy as "the psychotherapeutic use of movement toward physical and psychic integration of the individual (American Dance Therapy Association (ADTA), 1986, p. 1). Ganet-Sigel (1986) described it as a psychotherapeutic approach that focuses on the use of movement as the medium of change. "By working with muscular patterns and focusing on the interrelationships between psychological and physical processes, patients are helped to experience, identify, and express feelings and conflicts" (Ganet-Sigel 1986, p. 1). Using kinesthetic and visceral modalities, patients release emotional and physical blocks stored in the body that are often a beginning to relieving stress and anxiety. As patients reveal emotions and develop clearer understandings of their revelations, they can explore the use of alternative behaviors and work towards becoming healthier and better functioning individuals (Ganet-Sigel, 1986).

What processes are used in dance/movement therapy? This approach to therapy relies primarily on the use of body movement to express feelings that patients may have difficulty verbalizing. Using a combination of nonverbal kinesthetic movement and verbal therapy, clients begin to develop an awareness of unconscious material that is expressed during movement. After movement, clients talk and put words to the feelings that emerged during movement and to issues triggered by the movement such as a past memory or different type of association. As they become able to look at and listen to their unconscious (as revealed through their motoric expression), a different and deeper level of awareness develops. The therapist builds on what clients present. As client awareness deepens, the process of healing and the development of adaptive functioning emerges. Dance/movement has helped patients reveal past traumas, replace maladaptive social behaviors, and reintegrate lost or wounded portions of their psyche.

Dance/movement therapy is not a new discipline. In June of 1942, Marian Chace began using it with psychotic patients at St. Elizabeth's Hospital in Washington, DC and the positive effects of movement on patients were observed. For many years, it was recognized primarily on the East and West coast as an alternative approach to treating the severely ill psychotic patient. However, after earning her certificate as a registered dance/movement therapist in 1972, Jane Ganet-Sigel expanded awareness of this field when she opened a private practice and later started a graduate program in the study of dance/movement therapy at Columbia College in Chicago in 1982. This book is a chronicle of her struggle and success in bringing dance/movement therapy to the Midwest, her therapeutic work with outpatient clients, and an exploration of the instructional approach she used to train aspiring dance/movement therapists. The authors describe how Ganet-Sigel's belief in human beings' fundamental desire to realize health can lead them to express repressed feelings through the movement process. This book is recommended for therapists, educators, and dancers who are interested in the use of movement as a means to discovering intrapsychic understanding and healing.

Both the medical community and lay society are giving greater attention to alternative forms of therapeutic treatment as people become more aware of the power of the mind-body connection and as the line between purely physical illness and emotional problems dissolves (Lewis, 1986). As these treatment modalities become apparent, the academic community's responsibility to make new knowledge available also becomes evident. In recognition of these important therapeutic advancements, this book focuses on a field that has played a significant role in advancing our knowledge about the mind-body connection, dance/movement therapy. *The Art and Practice of Dance/Movement Therapy* offers therapeutic, educational, and historical information about the pioneering efforts of one person who has shaped the practice and training of dance/movement therapy, as well as creative arts therapists and related therapies. This book fills a gap in the field about the emergence of dance/movement therapy as an alternative treatment modality for clients who suffer from mental health problems. What makes Ganet-Sigel's work significant is her artistry as a teacher and a clinician, her facility to translate theory into practice and practice into theory. Students will find this text useful to their own professional development and appreciate others' experiences that portray the perils and pitfalls of many novice therapists.

Many hours of a related research study are also presented in this book. The findings reported were obtained using the following processes. Thirty-six individuals including students, colleagues, former clients, friends, and family members were interviewed for this textbook. Of this group, 18 therapists including 2 psychiatrists, a psychologist, 10 dance/movement therapists, 2 psychodrama therapists, a psychiatric social worker, an art and a music therapist responded to questions. The demographics of the interview group were as follows: 26 females, and 10 males; 31 Caucasians, 3 African-Americans, 1 Hispanic, and 1 Asian-American.

After obtaining an informed consent, participants were asked to respond to a semi-structured interview protocols. Questions for the clients focused on learning how the process of dance/movement therapy helped them become healthy. They were asked to describe: (a) the issue/problem that brought them to work with Ganet-Sigel, (b) why they chose dance/movement therapy (c) how their work with Ganet-Sigel changed their personal sense of self, created a sense of well-being, brought about fundamental deep internal changes or otherwise influenced the quality of their lives, (d) what specific aspects of dance/movement therapy helped to facilitate these changes, (e) how the process of dance/movement therapy facilitated these changes, and (f) how their work with Ganet-Sigel influenced their lives.

Questions for students centered on learning how Ganet-Sigel facilitated students' ability to transfer classroom learning into practice.

They were asked to describe: (a) why they chose to study dance/movement therapy, (b) the methods or ways in which Ganet-Sigel teaches, (c) how Ganet-Sigel helped them make the connections between theory, textbook readings, and actually working with a client, (d) the ways in which positive learning experiences were provided, and (e) the feelings they had while they were Ganet-Sigel's students.

Questions for colleagues focused on obtaining other professionals' points of view about the dance/movement therapeutic process. They were asked to describe: (a) the nature of their relationship with Ganet-Sigel and (b) their perceptions of dance/movement movement therapy in general as well as (c) their perceptions regarding the nature of Ganet-Sigel's work.

Questions for friends and family centered on learning about Ganet-Sigel as an individual and woman. They were asked to: (a) characterize the nature of their relationship with Ganet-Sigel, and (b) discuss how Ganet-Sigel's life changes, her quest to become a dance/movement movement therapist, and her work as a dance/movement therapist influenced the nature of their relationship with her.

Each interview was audio-taped and transcribed by a graduate student in education. The transcripts were sent back to the interviewees accompanied by a letter that asked them to read the manuscript, check the accuracy, write in any necessary revisions and return them to the first author. Corrections were made to the transcripts as appropriate prior to the data analysis phase.

Data was analyzed inductively guided by Spradley's (1980) scheme of domain analysis and by the constant-comparative method proposed by Glaser and Strauss (1967). Domain analysis worksheets were created to organize interviewee responses from protocols into categories. A dependability audit was conducted on each transcript with a graduate student in education to assure the validity of the domains.

Included in this book are vignettes of actual work with patients, an overview of Ganet-Sigel's teaching strategies, and biographic information that provides an integrated analysis of how dance/movement therapy has become an important approach to healing the mind and body. An analysis of each case study offers insight into how dance/movement therapy has been used to help clients make fundamental and healthy changes, in many cases where verbal therapy did not bring about sustained healing. The instructional strategies Ganet-Sigel has used to help students translate textbook concepts and classroom learning into a process of becoming a therapist are explicated. The interplay between the professional and personal lives of a therapist and life experiences that have influenced Ganet-Sigel's development as a therapist are also described.

Ganet-Sigel's pioneering efforts to heighten awareness of the field, as well as her courage to enter into a profession at a time when women of her era typically remained at the home and cared for their children and husbands, is a remarkable story about leadership, love, and commitment. A chronicle of Ganet-Sigel's seminal work as the first registered dance/movement therapist in the Midwest, a founding member of the American Dance/Movement Therapy Association, and Chair of one of the five accredited programs in the nation is an important epoch in the field that has yet to be told. In a general context, she serves as a leader among women.

A child psychiatrist shared that:

> Observing Jane work gave me the opportunity to witness a remarkable therapeutic environment. By establishing a form of mutual communication through movement, Jane was able to entice an autistically withdrawn child from a private world into ours. This feat was beyond our usual mode of verbal communication. Hope for future development began with this breakthrough into shared experience. This is where the real treatment of these withdrawn children could begin. *Glorye Wool, M.D.*

A psychiatrist who specializes in the treatment of adults observed that:

> Dance/movement therapy directly connected with the person's innermost experiences and feelings and was able to impact on them through that deep connection which was not accessible oftentimes through talking or listening or something that wasn't physical. Through movement, the client is able to connect with their innermost and deepest feelings . . . and through Jane's therapeutic understanding, Jane can help the client change . . . there's a physical connection through the movement therapy to the client's experiences: somatic and emotional experiences. And through that physical connection, the person's emotions and somatic experiences can be changed actually.
>
> *Jack S. Pierce, M.D.*

A dancer, choreographer, and educator stated that:

> Healing the whole self has to involve healing the body. All of life's unresolved trauma are memories locked in our tissue, muscles, and viscera as well as in our mind and spirit. In order to heal the whole self, you have to also heal the body. People who are seriously trying to heal themselves need to heal through the body and dance/movement therapy is the field that is aimed at doing that.
>
> *Nana Shineflug, Founder and Artistic Director of the Chicago Moving Company and Faculty in the Departments of Theater and Interdisciplinary Arts. Columbia College, Chicago, IL.*

A fellow creative arts therapist commented that:

> Jane Ganet-Sigel is one of the pioneers in dance/movement therapy. She has not only influenced that field but creative arts therapies in general. Her contributions to the training of new clinicians is invaluable. Her work will influence the development of the field for years to come.
>
> *Roseann Kasayka, PhD, RMT-BC Music Therapist*

As Ganet-Sigel enters retirement, this book will likely become a key text for educators and therapists who work in schools, hospitals, clinics, and private practice and are considering alternative treatment modalities for the difficult to reach client. For professors of dance/movement therapy, this book can become an important text-book in influencing program development and helping teachers learn how to train students in the "process" of becoming a therapist. For dancers and choreographers, dance/movement therapy provides a showcase of how artistic expression may be facilitated through the strengthening of the mind/body connection.

PART I

THE THEORY AND PRACTICE OF DANCE/ MOVEMENT THERAPY

Introduction

In the opening chapter of this textbook, the authors discuss the theoretical conceptions of dance/movement therapy and describe how theory can be used to guide practice. Next they present Ganet-Sigel's theoretical framework and illustrate how it guided her approach to the treatment of clients. In Chapter two, following a brief biographical account, the authors recount Ganet-Sigel's pioneering efforts to bring dance/movement therapy to private practice, psychiatric hospitals, and geriatric centers in the Midwest and Chicago. They also describe her early collaborations with other health providers. Despite Ganet-Sigel's occasionally difficult journey while introducing dance/movement therapy to medically trained therapists, she relied upon her belief in the healing powers of this approach and an unfettered vision. The authors provide an overview of her work as a program developer and describe how she encouraged medical professionals to question their long-standing philosophies. In chapter three, the authors describe Ganet-Sigel as a teacher through the eyes of her students. Based upon interviews with current and former students, the authors illustrate how she used teaching strategies and humor to provide leadership, mentorship, and training to over 150 of nearly 1,500 of the dance therapists who are currently registered in the American Dance Therapy Association of the United States. In chapter four, based upon client interviews, the authors describe how Ganet-Sigel has successfully treated patients in an outpatient setting.

CHAPTER 1

Theoretical Approaches and Techniques in Dance/Movement Therapy

Guiding Questions

1. *Why is it important for the dance/movement therapist to have a theoretical framework?*
2. *In what ways can theory be used in the development of a treatment plan?*
3. *How can effort/shape analysis be used to guide the therapists' assessment of a client's issues?*
4. *What are the major tenets that comprise Ganet-Sigel's theoretical approach?*
5. *In what ways has Ganet-Sigel applied theory in her work with clients?*

. . . And when [Jane] described her work with children, the physical work, the movement, and so on, this was very, very understandable to me. And I could see that she was a person [who] approached the whole idea of therapy in a way that was similar to mine. It was very close to the earth, very much understanding that everybody's basic need was for closeness, emotional and physical closeness. It starts the other way around. It starts with physical closeness which then gets translated into what an infant understands as emotional or experiences as emotional.

Mildred Lachmann-Chapin, ATR

In this chapter, the authors: (1) describe why it is important for dance/movement therapists to identify their theoretical dispositions, (2) describe techniques that they may use in their work, (3) illustrate how theory can be used with an actual client, and (4) offer a process model for establishing a therapeutic relationship. This chapter begins with a discussion of the following questions. What is theory? Why is theory important to the aspiring dance/movement therapist? How can theory be used to guide the development of treatment objectives and the therapeutic process? Next the authors provide a brief discussion about how effort/shape analysis can be used to assess the client's movement. After describing Ganet-Sigel's theoretical framework, they discuss the theory that Ganet-Sigel has practiced throughout her career while working with emotionally disturbed children and adults in private practice. Next they illustrate how theory can be applied in working with an actual client. Finally, they offer a process model to describe how the therapist begins to establish a therapeutic alliance with clients.

What Is Theory?

Theory is the expression of beliefs, a symbolic construction that helps systematize generalizable facts or laws, as well as a means for noting relationships among facts, concepts, components, or variables (Macdonald, 1995; Snow, 1973). Theory provides a mechanism for clarifying the nature of concepts or problems. However, the validation of theory rests primarily on logic and values, rather than empirical support (Ornstein & Hunkins, 1998).

Whether or not consciously acknowledged by the dance/movement therapist, theory is part of therapeutic decision-making. An awareness of theory is essential to becoming an effective practitioner. Although some dance/movement therapists may consider it to be rather impractical, without a theoretical framework, it may be difficult to fully comprehend the dynamics of clients' movements,z render a thorough assessment of observed movement, articulate treatment goals, or implement appropriate dance/movement techniques. Rather than being a mere technician, the dance/movement therapist can use theoretical knowledge for the practical purpose of explaining, prescribing, generalizing, and describing what kinds of treatment approaches are most suitable in working with specific client populations.

By having a clear understanding of theory, the dance/movement therapist is likely to be more skilled in analyzing and synthesizing his/her observations of clients' movements, organizing impressions and assessments of their particular maladies, and recommending comprehensive treatment plans. Engaging in thinking and talking about theory encourages dance/movement therapists to ask "how" and "why" questions about what they observe. The skilled dance/movement therapist recognizes that an understanding of theory provides specialized lenses through which to see, think, and know; it connects philosophical knowledge to ways of analyzing, knowing, and appreciating the clients' experiences in practice-based settings.

Theory does not necessarily suggest a prescribed action. Instead theory helps the therapist to view the patterns inherent to a set of events or phenomena and organize seemingly unconnected impressions. Theory can aid in making sense of observations that might at first appear confusing so that logical impressions may coalesce. Through interpretation, criticism, and the location of specific patterns, powerful generalizations can be identified and used to aid in treatment planning. Theory can be helpful in understanding the reality of a client's malady, in explaining his/her movement, and in characterizing the nature of his/her interactions in the world.

The therapist needs theory as a foundation for establishing the type of practice and techniques that he/she will utilize. Understanding theoretical precepts embedded within specific models has implications for therapeutic practice and may be instructive in the development of treatment plans. In actual practice, the dance/movement therapist will employ methods and tools that complement the client's needs, therapeutic goals, and dynamics of his/her contextualized situation. Although it is important to distinguish between theory and technique, a therapist should select a theory (or components of multiple theories) to which he/she ascribes. However, the technique(s) that the therapist employs will depend much upon the nature of the clients' conflicts, symptomatology and ability/limitations. For example, consider how theoretical viewpoints may be differentially grounded as exemplified by the object relations model, the self-psychological model, and the ego-psychological model.

The object relations theorists including Kernberg (1976), Mahler (1968, 1975), and Masterson (1981) believe that psychic structures develop as the child constructs internal representations of self and others. Representations range from primitive to fantastic to relatively realistic and are associated with a wide range of effects such as fantasies and wishes. As the growing child struggles with these contradictory representations, feelings of self and others, he/she tends to split good and bad images into different representations. In mature individuals, these images are integrated into coherent representations of self and others accompanied by multiple complex qualities, which are selected and formed in part so that the individual is able to maintain an optimal measure of self-esteem, tolerable effects, and satisfaction of wishes (Perry, Cooper, and Michels, 1987). Healthy and adaptive functioning may emerge as the child internalizes a healthy bond between himself/herself and the primary maternal caregiver. However, any pattern that has been experienced with the primary maternal caregiver will re-emerge later in the individual's life. Damage during the early phases of child development lead to more severe problems such as psychosis, while damage that occurs in the later phases of child development typically result in neurosis.

Self-psychological theorists such as Kohut (1971, 1977) Freed (1984), and Perry, Cooper, and Michels (1987) postulate that psychological structures of the self develop towards the realization of two classes of goals that are both innate and learned, the individual's ambitions and his/her ideals. Normal childhood development is characterized by the child's grandiose idealization of self and others, exhibitionistic expressions of strivings and ambitions, and the empathic responsiveness of parents and others to these needs. Under healthy conditions, the child's emergent skills, talents, and internalization of empathic objects lead to the development of a sturdy self and capacities for creativity, joy, and ongoing empathic relationships.

Ego psychological theorists including the Blancks (1994) and Winnicott (1965) emphasize the centrality of the ego in the development of a healthy and adaptive individual. Behavior is mediated by the ego. The ego is viewed as a defensive compromise among wishes and impulses, the inner conscience, self-observation, and criticism, and the potentialities as well as the demands of reality. For the client who may be suffering from childhood maladies, this information provides a framework for articulating treatment goals.

How might a dance/movement therapist who ascribes to the work of object-relations, self-psychological, and ego-psychological theorists use theoretical precepts in developing treatment goals for a client suffering from anorexia nervosa? Several ideas may be culled from these theories to help the therapist formulate questions about the client's level of functioning and the etiology of their illness. Using these theoretical ideas, the dance/movement therapist might ask how the client's early development may be impacting their current level of functioning. In trying to learn about the client's early development, the therapist will want to determine if the client has experienced deficits or lack of appropriate phase development that have given rise to the nature of the client's illness. The therapist might ask if there are any developmental deficits that interfere with the client's ability to function in the present day. The therapist will recognize that a client's need for nurturing may arise from a lack of good enough mothering or a holding environment. If a client is suffering from having experienced an unhealthy symbiosis, then through the therapeutic process, the dance-movement therapist will recapitulate the early symbiotic relationship. If the client suffers from confusion about his/her identity, movement techniques will be used to help the client get in touch with his/her body and develop a sense of autonomy.

Effort-Shape Analysis and Dance/Movement Therapy

Observing the clients' movements supplies cues with which the therapist must work. Effort-shape analysis utilizes a language to record or systematically analyze clients' movements that give credence to the therapist's observations. Effort shape analysis is a way of looking at movement and describing movement. Effort shape gives you the quality and a sense of the effort involved. This mode of observation also permits the dance/movement therapist to communicate with colleagues who are involved with the treatment of clients.

Effort is a system that describes the clients' movement in terms of how kinetic energy is used. The dynamics of effort can be observed along four motion factors: weight, time, space, and flow. Different effort qualities result from an inner attitude (conscious or unconscious). Each factor also has two dimensions: weight (firm, gentle), time (sudden, sustained), space (direct, flexible), and flow (bound, free) (Laban, 1971).[1] There are two levels of assessing the four factors, measurable and objective, and classifiable and subjective. For weight, time,

---

[1] The first dimension listed parenthetically reflects fighting; the second dimension reflects yielding.

space, and flow, the degree of resistance, speed, direction, and control respectively may be objectively measured. For weight, time, space, and flow, the degree of levity, duration, expansion, and fluency respectively may be classified or assessed subjectively. Each component can be expressed among eight differentiated patterns: *punch, slash, dab, flick, press, wring, glide,* and *float.*

According to Laban (1971):

> Weight, space, time, and flow are the motion actions towards which the moving person adopts a specific attitude. These attitudes can be described as:
>
> > a relaxed or forceful attitude towards weight,
> > a pliant or lineal attitude towards space,
> > a prolonging or shortening attitude towards time,
> > a liberating or withholding attitude towards flow.
>
> A specific combination of several of these eight elements of movement is observable in every action, and is most evident in the so-called basic actions in which the easily discernible factors of space, time, and weight are mainly considered (p. 76).

The analysis of body actions can be described by answering the following questions:

> (1) Which part of the body moves?
> (2) In which direction or directions of space is the movement exerted?
> (3) At what speed does the movement progress?
> (4) What degree of muscular energy is spent on the movement?
> *(Laban, 1971, p. 27).*

Each client's manner of movement is as individual as his/her signature. A client does not move with only one element. Effort reflects the client's inner drives or impulses from which movements emerge.

Shape is a system that describes the quality or actual form of movement as a client moves through space. Shape also can be used to characterize the client's relationship to the environment. Shape relates to the differentiation of the self from the object (Lewis, 1986). Three planes of shape have been identified by Lamb (1965): horizontal (side-to-side), vertical (up-down), and sagittal (forwards/backward) or length, breadth, and height respectively. Corresponding movement along these planes can be described as the spreading and enclosing, rising and descending, and advancing and retiring respectively. How are effort-shape components related? Lewis offers an example.

> If an individual exhibits a preponderance of efforts over shape, he will appear to be aloof, he may possess adequate drives but no ability to direct his need satisfaction to the appropriate object in the environment. He may have a somewhat-functioning ego, but he would be bereft of the capacity to relate to others (p. 165).

Conversely, if the individual demonstrates far more shaping than efforts, his relationship to his environment may lack feeling or reality-based sophistication. . . . (p. 165).

A discrepancy between space and weight efforts, shaping, and and/or time efforts is indicative of conflict behavior (Kestenberg & Lamb, Cited in Lewis, 1986, p. 165). When effort is appropriately matched with shape, skills in communications, presentation of self and ideas, and the observable manner in which one functions in daily life activities, then the individual, claimed Lamb (1965) is probably functioning more adaptively. Lamb also asserted that the degree to which ". . . a person can enlarge his/her repertoire, especially where posture and gesture are seen to overlap, the more he/she is thought to be acting in accordance with his real self" (Lamb, 1965, Cited in Lewis, 1986, p.167).

The dance/movement therapist observes clients' movements and recognizes specific efforts, quality, and habitual patterns. Awareness of the qualities of each client's movement patterns culled through these observations can be used to guide the enlargement of clients' repertoire of movement and to facilitate more adept movement from the inside out, not from the outside in. While not all dance/movement therapists use the effort-shape system to describe clients' movements, Mason (1974) suggested that effort-shape analysis could be used to bridge the gap between movement thinking and word thinking and bring about a deeper understanding of movement.

One goal of dance/movement therapy is to broaden clients' existing repertoires of adaptive choices and move them toward individuation. The therapist can utilize movement as a bridge between the conscious and unconscious world to draw those unconscious states into the realm of conscious reality. The therapeutic aim is to change the client's movement patterns based upon the belief that alterations in motoric behavior will lead to changes in inner attitudes, social behavior, and physiological responses.

The keys to understanding the rationale behind why individuals hold their muscles and thus their bodies in particular postures, why breathing is executed in various manners, why individuals move in certain patterns, and why illnesses effect particular physiologic organ systems all lie in personal histories which distribute, sculpt, and choreograph psychic energy (Lewis, 1986, pp. 138–139).

However as Weiner (1985) has observed

. . . resistance in the musculature parallels characterological fixations in the psychoanalytical sense. . . . The body is like a safety deposit box to which a person can go time and time again to tap into these early pleasurable excitations. It is the original cathexis of early relationships. The sublimation of these early relationships take place in rhythms, motion, *and* shape. . . . The emotional conflicts that may be connected to the cathexis are worked out or sustained through the polarities of moving, such as in contraction and release, fall and recovery, strength and flexibility, motion and stillness (p. 36).

How does pathology occur? Lewis suggested that

> If individuals do not have the appropriate internal and external environment to develop, phase-related maladaptive experiences get stored in the body. The specific muscular system or physiological organ in which these experiences are cathected depends on their actual or symbolic relationship to a person's development (p. 139).
>
> If the ego as mediator has insufficient boundaries or lacks sufficient development, the unconscious will flood consciousness. Psychic energy lacking ego assimilation and adaptation will fill the individual with the stuff of which myths and fairytales are made. Without relativization and humanization, external reality too becomes transformed into a fantastic world to be feared or perhaps to be overwhelmed by (p. 139).

How can healing and recovery be manifest?

> . . . for the learning of a particular level in functioning to take place, the individual must not only have arrived at a sufficient maturational level . . . organized all the past . . . and have progressed into a state of disequilibrium (Lewis, 1986, p .141).

Additionally, the environment must be appropriate to the conditions necessary for clients to fully integrate a higher level of functioning, but he/she must also be in an adequate and appropriate environment which has all the necessary elements in order for learning to occur. The therapist also plays a central role in influencing the clients' recovery. He/she must be able to discern the client's pattern of movement by moving in and out of the role of observer, analyzer, empathizer, and leader (North, 1995). Yet at the same time, the therapist must provide the client with the necessary space, timing, and pacing to facilitate self-discovery. Naturally the therapist's capacity for intervention will require a foundation in movement approaches and making informed responses to the client's movement manifestations, an understanding of the client's presenting problems, and an evolving assessment of the client's capacity for dipping into potentially charged emotional content.

Just knowing theory or having an intellectual understanding of therapeutic techniques does not necessarily make an individual an effective therapist. How can one assess the effectiveness of a therapist? What are the characteristics of an effective therapist? Table 1.1 highlights the differences between the intentional (effective) and ineffective therapist across the following domains: (a) theoretical dispositions, (b) use of interventions, (c) observation, (d) analysis of clients' issues, (e) professionalism, and (f) ethics.

Table 1.1. CHARACTERISTICS OF THERAPISTS

	INTENTIONAL	INEFFECTIVE
Theoretical dispositions	Has an identifiable theoretical framework that guides practice	Lacks an understanding of theory; practice is not grounded in any theoretical precepts
Use of interventions	Matches techniques to clients' observed behaviors and presenting issues	Uses interventions idiosyncratically, irrespective of clients' needs
Observation	Uses a systematic approach to observing clients' movement repertoire	Assesses clients' movement intuitively, avoids the use of systematic observations
Analysis of clients' issues	Listens to and observes clients attentively and objectively	Listens selectively to clients and formulates an impression of client's issues without adequate evidence
Professionalism	Provides a supportive, compassionate and empathic therapeutic environment; respects the dignity and individuality of each client	Provides a therapeutic environment that is grounded in the therapist's needs and emotional issues. Is judgmental about client's issues.
Ethics	Maintains client confidentiality	Is ignorant of and disrespectful about the need to maintain client confidentiality

Ganet-Sigel's Theoretical Framework

What is dance/movement therapy? According to the American Dance Therapy Association (1986), it is "The psychotherapeutic use of movement toward the physical and psychic integration of the individual" (ADTA Manual, 1986, p. 1). It is a form of psychotherapy that focuses on the use of movement as a medium of change. "By working with muscular patterns and focusing on the interrelationships between psychological and physiological processes, clients are helped to experience, identify and express feelings and conflicts" (Ganet-Sigel, 1986, p. 1). Ganet-Sigel relates dance/movement therapy to the "3-R's"–dance/movement therapy releases, reveals, and reconstructs. From this kinesthetic and visual modality, individuals and groups are helped to release emotional and physical blocks stored in the body, often a beginning to relieving stress and anxiety; and to reveal emotional issues, through symbolic representation, images, memories, fantasies, and personal situations from their life experience. With a clearer sense of self awareness, alternative modes of behavior can be explored and a reconstruction of behavior will allow for a healthier functioning person.

Two terms, "dance" and "movement" therapy, are used to describe the profession. Many conversations ensued about changing the title of this therapeutic approach. At one point, dance was later modified to movement by those who wished to detach themselves from dance as a performing art. The word "dance" in our culture has a more narrow definition. However Chace liked the phrase, "dance therapy" because using dance in the title, she believed connoted the expressiveness associated with dance. In contrast, others believed that in the past, stereotypes associated with the word dance caused some misunderstanding when it was used in the context of the phrase "dance therapy." As a result, the phrase "dance/movement therapy" was coined to replace the former description and to clarify the purpose of this treatment modality. There is also some variation among dance/movement therapists in their use of music in treatment. Those who make little or less use of the music itself but instead rely on the internal rhythms developed by the patient in response to the music more frequently use the term "movement." However, the rhythmic quality of movement, particularly as related to groups, and concepts of space, time, force, and balance have roots in dance itself. Many believe it important to maintain identification with dance as an art form, for it is that balance between art and science that makes the creative and therapeutic use of dance so valid and successful. However as in all disciplines, understanding the concepts generally tends to prove more helpful than depending upon the name.

The use of dance/movement therapy as an intervention that is grounded in the belief that the soma and the psyche are interrelated whereby cognitive awareness affects responses in the body and what is happening with the tension and relaxation in the muscular systems affects body-image and self esteem. In this sense, the body and mind are seen as having equally important and reciprocal influences in totality of an individual's functioning. Every thought, activity, memory, fantasy or image involves some degree of muscular reaction and felt tension. The body itself is a container for memories as well as a source for responding and learning. One of the primary roles that dance/movement therapists fulfill is clarifying the importance of the body, not only in its relationship to emotions and learning, but also its accuracy as a communicative force.

All life is made up of movement. Our very existence is made up of both voluntary and involuntary sensory-motor responses to inner sensations and the environment without. We are continually acting upon these impressions. Even when we are "still," experimental evidence suggests that muscular tension can be localized to particular muscle groups so that energy is released in sufficient amount to be measured, even in the thinking processes (Kestenberg, 1995). Life initially is represented by tactile, thermal, and pain impressions which are acted upon by motor activity. While in infancy, the child's movement begins as random and uncoordinated. As a child matures, he/she is better able to control his gross motor activities. Adults heed and respond to the body communication of the infant. As the child acquires the capacity for language and begins to communicate verbally those around him/her tend to place less significance upon his/her physical responses. The child's capacity for verbal communication processes receives greater recognition and acknowledgment, while the non-verbal expressions may receive less and less acknowledgment. Slowly as the child evolves, communication is perceived to be comprised mostly if not solely by language.

The bond that an infant may develop within the first few months of life is critical to his/her latter development, for it is during this period that faulty concepts may develop. The child's kinesthetic sense begins during the vital pre-verbal mother-child interaction. Healthy bonding manifests when the infant develops a basic trust through the ease in which the infant moves through and from "oneness" with mother to "individual." (Erickson, 1950, Mahler, 1968, 1975). From birth to six weeks the child is in limbo, bridging the space between two environments, from womb to mother's and father's arms; the newborn has no past and no psychology. The infant enters the world with "unique inherited potential" and a biological readiness that will allow him/her to receive what the world offers.

The comfortable predictability with which the mother responds to the infant's inner work is the beginning of social trust. The unfamiliar sights, odors, sounds, temperatures and movements enter the infant's environments and the dialogue with life begins with his/her own gestures, fragmented movements "with" one another, at which time the child's space is enclosed, enlarging as he/she moves from oneness to separateness. As the child looks, sucks, grasps, reaches with mouth and eyes, flaps arms and legs, he/she comes into contact with an environment, that hopefully he/she will perceive is a friendly and a comforting one. The infant begins to sense his/her boundaries. As the infant develops he/she reaches out and creeps away, returns to home-base, checking in with mother for positive refueling, then moves away again, possibly a little further. The search for autonomy begins. The child receives positive or negative reinforcement by what is mirrored in the faces of those who look at him/her. Movement at this stage involves holding on and letting go repeatedly.

The constancy with which the child is responded to in his/her disappearances and reappearances, tensions and relaxation, acting and reacting must be also be accompanied by firm reassurance. The child's inability to hold on and let go with discretion must be safeguarded by an encouraging environment. The encouragement "to stand on his/her own feet" must protect him against "shame and early doubt."

The upright child now moves out into space clinging, pushing away, shadowing, darting away as he/she gradually claims his/her body. Under conditions of oppression, a child may remain a child forever. There must be constant translation of child's inner and outer explosions into comprehensive ordinary human emotions like hope and anger and courage to go on when adversity strikes. Subsequently, the person can then walk, run, climb, jump, leap, start and stop, and identify a self in a good relationship with the outer world. The establishment of trust through the synchrony of mother-child is the beginning of a harmonious journey through the sequence of psychosexual and psychosocial development.

Movement helps the evolving child by facilitating his/her acquaintance with his/her own boundaries and capacity and his/her relationship to the outer world. We do not know very much about the body unless we move it. Movement provides a mechanism to unite different parts of our body. Through movement, the child develops a definitive relationship to the outside world and to the object. As the child makes contact with the outside world, he/she is able to correlate the diverse impressions concerning his/her own body. The knowledge of one's body, to a great extent, is dependent upon our action. The postural model of the body is a creation and a construction and not a gift; it has to be built up.

Posture is one aspect of body image. Movement has the potential to catalyze changes in body image. As visceral changes become felt experiences, kinesthetic sensations such as the articulation of body parts, recognition of bodily sensations such as breathing, or awareness of muscular activity, can contribute to the patient's recognition and development of body image (Sandel, Chaiklin & Lohn, 1993). Mahler's work (1968, 1975) on emotional development or "psychological birth" lends support to the premise that there must be a recognition of the self as a separate physical entity before the individuation process can successfully occur. At the onset, the infant has no boundaries; internal and external are interchangeable. He/she is an extension of the mother's body (Liebowitz, 1992). As the growing infant begins to discriminate between his/her own body and that of his/her mother, if healthy development takes place, then a sense of separateness and individuation is achieved (Mahler, 1968). The images we develop of ourselves affects and is affected by all our perceptions, experiences, and actions. A man or woman who perceives himself as insecure and vulnerable will move differently from one who perceives himself to be strong. Likewise, if a child is treated as though he/she was inept, his body image would incorporate these feelings along with his/her reactions to other people's impressions and to his own. Schilder (1950) writes:

> The postural model of our body is connected with the postural models of the bodies of others. There are connections between the postural models of fellow human beings. We experience the body images of others. Experience of our body image and experience of the bodies of others are closely interwoven with each other. Just as our emotions and actions of others are inseparable from their bodies (p. 16).

Motion influences body image and can bring about a change in the psychic attitude. This relationship, the connection between movement change and psychological change in dance/movement therapy, becomes evident when as a result of movement intervention a client who has successfully worked through feelings of a distorted body image, also experiences a change in his/her own psychic attitude.

Emotional awareness develops as individuals recognize and interpret the motoric actions of others. Emotional responses to other people usually arise from our interpretations of the bodily actions and reactions of others as they are experienced through kinesthetic recognition. Kinesthetic empathy, which occurs mostly on an unconscious level, contributes to the verbal and nonverbal communication between people. The position of the body, gesturing movement, and breathing patterns are a few examples of movement behavior that can be examined within the framework of expressive movement. Qualitatively the way in which individuals move, the range of their movement, and visceral energy that accompanies movement, rather than the static positioning, reflects their expressions.

There are many types of situations that can stimulate emotional responses. Consider the sadness that is evoked when one loses a friend, or joyfulness that is experienced by the parents who have witnessed the healthy birth of their newborn. Emotions can also be felt when we perceive another's emotional state such as remembering or imagining being trapped in an elevator. Contagiously experiencing illness or fear as demonstrated by an actress can evoke a vicarious experience of someone else's fantasy state. In a related manner, the therapist can use imagery, action, and theme to help patients crystallize and integrate both physiological and psychological responses.

Imagery is just one of many techniques used in dance/movement therapy. However as therapeutic work commences it is essential that the dance/movement therapist and patient formulate treatment goals based on the needs of the individual patients or the group members. Developing treatment plans also requires that the therapist recognize that what is reasonable and appropriate for one patient may be too complicated or inappropriate for another. The individual remains the primary focus during therapy, whereas the processes inherent to dance/movement therapy provide tools to bring about healing.

Although dance therapists may ascribe to different theoretical models, the concepts of dance/movement therapy identified by Chace seem to be universal among many therapists (Chaiklin, 1975). She postulated four basic concepts: body action, symbolism, therapeutic movement relationship, and rhythmic group activity, which laid the foundation upon which to build a theory of dance/movement therapy. Chace was influenced by Sullivan (1953) who is credited with creating a new viewpoint, the interpersonal theory of psychiatry.

Sullivan suggested that personality is "the relatively enduring pattern of recurrent interpersonal situations which characterize a human life" (1953, p. 111). Claiming that personality is a hypothetical entity, he asserted that an individual does not and can not exist apart from his/her relations with others. From birth onward, the individual remains a member of a social field. Rather than deny the influence of heredity and maturity, Sullivan claimed that the distinct humanity of an individual results from social interactions (Hall & Lindzey, 1998). Moreover, physiological and psychological functioning may be altered by personal experiences in such a way that the individual biological status gives way to becoming a social organism. Rather than consisting of intrapsychic events, personality is thought to consist of interpersonal events. Personality serves a dynamic center of processes such as dynamisms, personifications and cognitive processes which occur in a series of interpersonal fields. Dynamisms, personifications, and cognitive processes are not the sole constituents of personality, they represent the major distinguishing structural features of Sullivan's theory (Hall & Lindzey, 1998).

Dynamisms are considered to be much like habits. A new feature can be added to a pattern without changing it so long as it is not significantly different from existing features. Most dynamisms serve the purpose of satisfying an individual's basic needs (Hall & Lindzey, 1998). Personifications emerge from a complex of feelings, attitudes, and conceptions embedded in experiences that are filled with self-satisfaction and/or anxiety. They are images that an individual has of himself/herself or others. When an infant is nursed and cared for by his/her mother, he/she develops a personification of a good mother. Other personifications are rarely accurate descriptions; they are formed to cope with others in isolated interpersonal circumstances and usually are quite influential in the development of attitudes towards others.

Sullivan's unique contribution about cognition as it relates to the development of personality is his classification of the prototaxic, parataxic, and syntaxic modes of experience. Prototaxic experiences may be thought of as: ". . . discrete series of momentary states of the sensitive organism (Sullivan, 1953, p. 29) similar to what James, Mandler, and Johnson-Laird (cited in Pickering and Skinner, 1990) has referred to as the "stream of consciousness." In the first few months of life, the prototaxic experience can be found in its purest form (Hall & Lindzey, 1998). The prototaxic modes consist of seeing casual relationships between events that occur proximately, but are not logically related. Sullivan believed that the thinking ability of most individuals does not advance beyond the parataxic mode. The highest mode of thinking, the syntaxic, consists of consensually validated symbols. Words and numbers are examples of consensually validated symbols which are agreed to have a standard meaning according to a group of people. "The syntaxic mode produces logical order among experiences and enables people to communicate with one another" (Hall & Lindzey, 1998, p. 144).

Sullivan is also credited with suggesting his conception of the therapist as participant-observer. He argued that: "The crying need is for observers who are growing observant of their observing" (Sullivan, 1964, p. 27).

> The theory of interpersonal relations lays great stress on the methods of participant observation, and relegates data obtained by other methods to at most a secondary importance. This implies that skill in the face to face, or person to person psychiatric interview is of fundamental importance (Sullivan, 1950, p. 122).

Sullivan suggests that heredity provides certain capacities for receiving and elaborating experiences. The biological substratum for personality development is provided by heredity and maturation, while the culture operating through a system of interpersonal relations makes manifest abilities and actual performance (Hall & Lindzey, 1998). Rather than asserting that personality is unalterable and formed at any early age, Sullivan claimed that it is malleable and subject to change as the individual experiences new interpersonal situations.

By visually and kinesthetically intuiting the patient's movement expressions, Chace learned how to establish a therapeutic relationship on a movement level. Using her acuminate sensitivity and skills in service of understanding the patient's movement communications, she was able to embody the emotional content of the patient's behavior into her own movement responses. Kinesthetically, she communicated to the patient "I know how you feel" thereby establishing affective, empathetic interactions. By reenacting the essential constellation that characterized the patient's movement expression, Chace entered his/her world. As she recreated the patient's behavior in her own body, she was able to perceive what was possible and expand the interaction. She would deepen this interaction by doing similar, more expansive, or complementary movements that were introduced by the patient. Variously she would reflect, broaden or complete a patient's movement to convey that she understood his/her behavior. By mirroring a significant gesture at the right time, for only as long as the patient would accept it, Chace was able to establish trust. Through her acceptance and understanding, she facilitated patients' ability to communicate repressed ideas and feelings and to risk new experiences and relationships (Lewis, 1986).

Balint (1968) also has stressed the importance of staying and moving with the patient in silence with the aim of communication understanding. Concurring with this approach, Liebowitz (1992) emphasized the importance of the therapist's skills. In particular, she pointed out that the therapist's movements: ". . . tuning in to and reflecting the patient's movement qualities, rhythms, and phrasing which may be as minimal as a foot tapping, a breathing rhythm, a hand gesture, or the nod of the head" (p. 108) can communicate a gesture of being with the patient, that will ultimately will be accepted and lead to a strengthening of the therapeutic alliance.

Chace believed dance is communication. In her view, distortions of body shape and function were maladaptive responses to conflict and pain. When the emotions become distorted ". . . some people bind energy, limit the use of space, [discount] body parts or hold their breath, to guard against feelings such as guilt, aggression and sexuality. Others become hyperactive, exploding in time and space in response to real or imagined fears." (Sandel, Chaiklin, & Lohn, 1993, p. 77). Through her work with disturbed patients, Chace learned that because dance activities helped patients feel both relaxed and stimulated, they were then able to express their emotions more freely.

> Since muscular activity expressing emotion is the substratum of dance, and since dance is a means of stimulating and organizing such activity, . . . dance could be a potent means of communication for the reintegration of the seriously ill patient (Sandel, Chaiklin, & Lohn, 1993, p. 77).

As patients began to feel and acknowledge their visceral responses and recognize the consequences of their motoric actions, readiness for change developed. However, as Chace discovered, change only occurred when patients are ready. Over time the intricate connections between alterations in posture and shifts in psychic attitude became apparent to her (Sandel, Chaiklin, & Lohn, 1993). The therapist's role as a facilitator in assisting patients also became evident. As the therapist begins to understand the relationship between the patient's movement, dance, and emotional communication, the therapist can help the patient to enlarge his/her capacity for movement and enhance the patient's cognitive understanding of the meanings embedded in his/her movement patterns (Sandel, Chaiklin, & Lohn, 1993).

How does the movement of a dancer differ from the movement expressed by patients? Differences may be described across a variety of domains, the use of symbolic action, the use of movement, and symbolic communication. Whereas both the patient and the dancer use symbolic action to communicate emotions that may not be expressed in words, their intention and level of consciousness in selecting movements differ. Dancers may select from a repertoire of movements and objectively choose to portray grief, horror, exaggerated joy or sorrow, or uncensored frenzy to an audience. In contrast the patient who suffers from mental illness gives an expression to subjective and at times complex emotions, through his/her movement patterns, that otherwise could not be communicated through the use of language. In this realm, movement and dance offer both the mover and the observer an opportunity to participate in an interaction that transcends culture, race/ethnicity, age, gender, socio-economic status, and illness, because the symbols are universal (Sandel, Chaiklin, & Lohn, 1993).

For some patients who suffer from mental illness and are ill at ease with the use of language, such as schizophrenics, dance/movement may offer them the only medium to communicate and/or to be understood.

> The camouflage of the movement symbol makes it easier for these patients to express needs, feelings, and desires. In dance/movement therapy symbolism offers patients a means to recall, re-enact, and re-experience. . . . some problems that can be successfully resolved by working solely on a symbolic level. The dance/movement therapist's acceptance of patient's symbolic communications encourages the patient to further his/her symbolic expressions (Sandel, Chaiklin, & Lohn, 1993, p. 77).

As the dance therapist responds to these expressions and offers imagery or provides thematic content to guide movement, the therapist and patient formulate new symbolic interactions. The dance therapist utilizes the neuromuscular linkage shared by dance and emotional expressions to select appropriate dance images (Sandel, Chaiklin, & Lohn, 1993).

Every aspect of human life has felt sense of rhythm. Without the structure that rhythm provides activities such as speaking, walking, working, and playing would be chaotic. Each individual experiences a unique undulation that is characteristic of the ebb and flow of the rhythm of his/her breath. However a group who moves together seems to develop a unified breath and pulse. Rhythm can be experienced as a feeling of solidarity and emotional synergy among people. Although some individuals may have difficulty or a reluctance to follow the spatial design of a movement, when feelings are expressed in a shared rhythm, each member draws from the unified pool of energy and experiences a heightened sense of strength and security. By adding the rhythm to actions that emerge from patient's awareness, the shared symbolic rhythmic action among group members becomes more sharply focused. Chace recognized the fundamental importance of rhythm as a therapeutic tool for communication and body awareness (Sandel, Chaiklin, & Lohn, 1993).

Other techniques such as (1) kinesthetic empathy, (2), exaggeration, (3) transforming movement into communication, (4) developing themes into action, (5) attention to the interactional aspect, (6) tension discharge, and (7) transitional objects built into dance/movement therapy are based on Jungian, Adlerian, Gestalt, Psychoanalytic/Freud- ian, Developmental and Object Relations theories. A brief description of each technique follows.

Kinesthetic empathy   involves placing yourself in kinesthetic empathy with another and serves two important functions: it can give pertinent information about how someone else is feeling, and it can foster the development of rapport. In using kinesthetic empathy, one is able to get a sense of what another is feeling.

> Through *the use of kinesthetic empathy* (italics added) . . . the most severely disturbed psychotic, autistic, or organically disabled can begin to be engaged in an therapeutic object relationship which will gradually provide the needed elements for healthy development (Lewis, 1986, p. 143).

During this process, it is important to incorporate into your own body the same posture, muscular tension, breathing pattern, and body movement as the client. However, it is crucial to remain in empathy for only a short period of time. Otherwise the intensity of the emotional experience may be hard to shake off as it becomes incorporated into the therapist's body. Another area of difficulty may occur by projecting impressions, values, and judgments onto the other person rather than recognizing that the material that emerges may be your own. Kinesthetic empathy is useful as a way to make contact with extremely regressed nonverbal clients, as well as from patient to patient. Sharing the same movement pattern while working with them helps to establish the beginnings of a relationship. In a way that is similar to working with the autistic child; the therapist needs to pay attention to the client's need for spatial and emotional distance.

Exaggeration involves the recognition of a particular aspect of someone's movement behavior that catches our attention (e.g. a deliberate or controlled quality, quick and sudden movements of the hand, or a sunken and heavy feeling) and asking a client to exaggerate that particular movement. For example, after getting the client to notice this pattern first, the therapist may suggest exaggerating the movement so that the characteristic quality stands out more. The client can be asked to explore expressive or communicative aspects. On a movement level, the therapist can suggest that the client allow more feelings to emerge and to allow movement to go where it feels like going. It is also possible to take movement quality into a different part of the body to notice if there is a similar or different emotional response. The client can be directed to verbalize what that particular part of the body may be saying or what it wants to do. The therapist can also model exaggeration for the client by responding to the movement that he/she initiates. The therapist may respond to the patient's communication by expanding his/her movement (Liebowitz, 1992). If the patient is swinging his/her arm gently, the therapist may respond with a swinging of the arm that is swift, with large circling motion, and great energy.

Transforming Movement into Communication is utilized to take movements that are dysfunctional in nature, (e.g. self-stimulating, repetitive, or used to keep others away) and use them as a basis in which to engage the client in a movement interaction. In attempting to use this technique, it is important not to mimic the other person. What seems to work best are movements similar to the client's or ones that are in direct response to what the client is doing.

Developing Themes into Action Despite the client's best intentions, words sometimes cover over or get in the way of experiencing the full impact of a particular feeling or situation. Developing this material into a body expression often crystallizes and deepens awareness. In addition, there is sometimes a discrepancy between what one says and what one does. Nonverbal behavior is hard to conceal or change. As a result, it often pinpoints precisely what is occurring. Some other issues that can be developed on a movement level include resistance, passivity, cooperation, and being a leader or a follower.

Attention to the Interactional Aspect All of the techniques suggested require astute sensitivity to nonverbal communication. Subtle changes in body posture can often indicate changes or adjustments in relationships. In a verbal therapy session, it is particularly important to take note of which people share similar positions or move in synchrony (rhythm) with one another. People can use themselves physically to unconsciously block another person, cut off or interrupt nonverbal sequences, or change position to avoid being in a movement interaction with others. The nonverbal level can provide information regarding status, power, relationships, cohesiveness, rapport, conflict, defenses, and emotional expression.

Tension Discharge For people who are stiff or tense, working with movement helps to loosen up the uncomfortable or stiff body parts. This usually results in increased blood flow, deeper breathing, and release of tension. Sometimes vigorous shaking of body parts (such as pretending to shake off water or dust) will allow for a cathartic release.

Transitional Objects For some people, relating directly to others can be a painful or frightening experience. At these times, the use of inanimate objects can serve to connect group members. Moreover, transitional objects, such as scarves, balloons, stretch ropes, stretch cloths, puff balls, etc., can allow for direct expression of feelings when real feelings are too frightening. At this point, the patient often believes that the object possesses these feelings rather than himself/herself. However at some point the patient begins to realize that in fact these are actually his/her own feelings. This process is much like a little baby who is able to give up his/her "blankey," go out into the world, and stand on his/her own two feet.

Different qualities of movement can spark memories, feelings, just from enacting movement to words such as moving fast or slow, strong or heavy. Motion words such as like *punch* or *slash* can lead to energized movements that may evoke emotions. Contrary movement patterns can be catalyzed through the use of opposite words such as *float* or *sway* can used to bring about a "rest" or "recuperation" to ease the tension used. Equilibrating movement that might result from contrary movement also allows clients to experience a homeostasis. Engaging in these types of movement allows clients to really feel these elements. Clients might also be offered objects such as a pillow to punch or other transitional objects to help them experience the authentic movement. While it is important to ensure that clients remain safe during movement, punching a pillow rather than swinging a punch into the air permits an authentic feeling of punch and permits a feeling of release.

Authentic Movement Whitehouse (1986) is credited with introducing the concept of authentic movement. This technique may become manifest when individuals move in response to the various sensations they feel. Movements may be responses to experiences from their past, or to ". . . new experiences that are unfolding for the individual to embody and integrate into their personality" (Lewis, 1996, p. 102). Some therapists like Lewis incorporate chanting and verbal response from the therapist. While these actions are considered controversial by others, the use of this technique challenges the assumption that the movement component of therapy is primarily nonverbal. Ganet-Sigel doesn't utilize authentic movement per se or archetype analysis purported by Jungian therapists; instead she relies more heavily on the use of thematic improvisation.

Working with Children with Emotional Disturbances

Children with emotional disturbances often suffer a variety of maladies as a result of maladapative emotional and/or physical development. Consequently they often find it difficult to identify, distinguish, and use their bodies in a developmentally appropriate and coordinated manner. Although patients of any age who are disturbed have difficulty expressing themselves verbally or revealing their feelings, because issues may be repressed and stored in the viscera, children with these problems can benefit from movement. Additionally dance/movement therapy can provide a way of reaching these children who otherwise were unreachable. Children with emotional disturbance often suffer from distorted body-image and an inability to abstract and conceptualize on the most elementary level. Therefore much of Ganet-Sigel's work with preschoolers who were emotionally disturbed focused primarily on helping clients to establish their own body image, release pent up emotions through an appropriate activity, and develop into a physically coordinated human being. Processes were often directed at strengthening the child's self-concept at a pre-verbal level.

Working with these children, "the therapist strives to re-educate undeveloped or weakened areas in the child while also maintaining and educating age-adequate and healthy areas" (Rauskin, 1990, p. 56). Because these children may suffer from learning problems and underdeveloped psychomotor development, the sessions must be directed at helping the child discover the meaning of his/her movement through movement rather than words.

The body, involved in all emotional experiences and psychomotor tensions, has the capacity to reveal both feelings of security and lack of security. Through creative activities and rhythmic techniques, the body becomes better coordinated and a new awareness of using the body on a conscious level develops. Therapeutic encounters foster the receipt of satisfying experiences that bolster feelings of confidence, which are so often lacking in these children. A new sense of pride is felt through new achievements. One of the goals of creative dance, or expressive movement, or dance/movement therapy, is to build a sufficient awareness of self, provide a mechanism that will bring about self-satisfying experiences, and promote adaptive functioning, rather than encourage the development of a professional dancer. Because these children exhibit a strong need for structure, movements often begin with boundaries narrower than might be age-appropriate to provide the children with optimal support and a sense some of security. The therapist provides external structures to assist clients whose intrapsychic vulnerability and ego dysfunction require a high degree of security and predictability. To avert the possibility of overwhelming or flooding the ego, the therapist must be sensitive to the client's level of frustration tolerance, and the need for resting periods to reduce the escalation of dysfunctional behaviors. Thus, the therapeutic process is molded and shaped around the needs of the client, responsive to his/her capacity for growth, while the degree of environmental structure ebbs and flows as the client's ego system is able to maintain itself.

In her early career, Ganet-Sigel worked with boys and girls between the ages of three and seven. The clients attended an out-patient program for emotionally disturbed children in the Therapeutic Nursery School at Chicago Read Mental Health Center in the State of Illinois. Dance/movement therapy was one component of a total treatment program staffed by the teachers, social workers, psychologists, a consulting psychiatrist, a speech therapist, child care workers, and a program director. The classroom activities were comprised of a number of therapeutically-oriented experiences. Even though there was tremendous freedom in class, children were given well defined limits of expected behavior and a loosely organized instruction in the use of the body.

To learn more about the children's level of motoric functioning, the Child Development Center's Psychoeducational Evaluation of Motor Abilities was administered to twenty-one children whose ages ranged from four to eleven. This test was devised by the staff because they believed there was a correlation between a child's poor body image and dysfunctioning motor abilities. The following areas were evaluated: (1) self-awareness and body concept, (2) balance, (3) spatial orientation, (4) locomotive skills (rolling, crawling, sitting, etc.), and (5) general coordination and visual motor activities. The following behavior areas were also evaluated: (1) general characteristics, (2) language and thought, (3) intrapersonal behavior, (4) problem behavior, and (5) interpersonal behavior. Based on the results of the study, the staff discovered that 75% of the children were functioning significantly below the average for their age group in all categories. This information was helpful in providing a baseline of the children's current motoric capacity and in establishing treatment goals.

Because of limited expressive and receptive language abilities, the children's communication often had to be interpreted by others. To build the children's self confidence, the dance/movement therapist used a careful balance of encouragement and limit setting. Initially the movement process was aimed at the development of large locomotion movements such as *walk, run, skip, leap, jump, hop, slide, gallop,* and *stride.* Non-locomotive movements such as *swings, bends, twists, stretch, rock, sway, push, pull, dodge, fall, crawl, roll, sit, lift,* and *strike,* were also stressed. During the movement process, an awareness of rhythms, beats, accents, beginning and stopping of music was introduced. Directions, timing, force, use of space, and quality of movement (soft, light, hard) were other aspects in which Ganet-Sigel helped children to become cognizant. Dealing with reality is important with children who suffer from severe emotional disturbance, because most of their lives are filled with too much fantasy.

How does the dance/movement therapist initiate interaction with these children? The therapist meets the class each time at the level of mood in which the children arrive, whether it be over active, quick changes of mood, aggressive, or depressed. The classroom curriculum is never comprised by a structured plan for any day. Instead each child's own interpretation is always accepted; the child is accepted as he/she is. Each child is given favorable support and reinforcement for what he does by the therapist's actions. These actions are either verbal approval or a non-verbal imitation of the child to show approval. There are no failures or bad movements. The therapist produces an environment that reduces failure. For example, the slightest movement or action is always noticed. During group sessions with up to four children, the therapist may focus on one child at one moment, however, he/she must always be aware of what is going on with the feelings, needs, frustrations, or angers taking place with the others in the class and respond accordingly.

During movement many pleasurable feelings may be awakened. The therapist is also alert to the over excited or panicky child whose emotions are becoming frightening and alternate from the creative to the structured. The child has multisensory experiences. Verbal response usually accompanies movements to designate body parts. Anything that happens in the room is creatively used as a learning experience.

Every activity with balloons, scarves, ropes, or anything else that happens along with the movement helps the child develop an awareness of both inner and outer space. These objects are used to help the child discover tensions of the body, relationship to objects, to self, control of different parts of the body, as well as relations to space, to environment, and to stimulate tactile experiences.

The therapist must not be afraid of merging with the child. Above all, the therapist must be authentic and respond honestly to his/her own feelings and those of the children. Non-verbal activities, verbal communication, and group integration served as a framework to offer therapeutic experiences that were used to stimulate self awareness among children with emotional disturbance.

Working with Clients in Private Practice

Ganet-Sigel's treatment of clients is supported by several fundamental beliefs. First, concurring with (Chodorow, 1995), she asserts that: "Emotion affects motion which affects emotion. Since the mind and body are engaged in reciprocal interaction, whatever the inner self experiences becomes manifest in the body. Correspondingly experiences in the body influence the inner self" (Ganet-Sigel, 1986). Second, she believes that despite individuals' diagnoses, symptoms, or maladies, all clients suffer from three basic conflicts: trust in humanity, issues that center around self-esteem, and a difficulty in seeing how they function in this world.

Working with clients in the context of their current reality, she remains empathic and thoughtful throughout the therapeutic process. Therapy begins as clients share their perceptions about present day and past experiences with her. During the movement session and based on her observation of clients' movement patterns or their own statements, Ganet-Sigel selects a theme that is consonant with clients' emotional state, (such as "let's work with the words *push* and *pull*") that she believes will initiate movement pattern. As she observes clients' movements with a second set of eyes and listens with a second set of ears and body, she interprets clients' movement patterns in relationship to the themes used. As clients start to reveal more about themselves, Jane helps them to reconstruct and understand the past. In subsequent sessions she selects different themes that might encourage the expression of other types of movement.

Later in the therapeutic process, after a trusting relationship has emerged, she will share her observations. She might ask the client: "Does that feel familiar? Are you aware that every time that I bring up this word or music that you hold your arm tight against your waist?" Gradually, Jane begins to help clients develop a conscious awareness of how the messages that they are conveying with their bodies may be heard or felt by others.

In her role, she offers clients an objective lens to view how they are currently different from the way they behaved in the past. When clients are revealing past traumas or conflicts that initially may have occurred at age five, Ganet-Sigel frequently tells them that unlike the past they have different ways to contend with difficult situations. She often reminds clients, "Today, you have the physical ability to fight back, the adult intelligence to cope differently, and the emotional maturity to understand the conflicts of the 5 year old so that now your behavior can be self-selected." Although she will tell clients that therapy does not erase or take away the pain of the past, she fervently believes that through the course of therapy clients develop better coping skills as the result of new understandings that evolve. As revised external and internal validity begins to emerge, clients are encouraged to use different and more adaptive responses.

Rather than try to determine the client's diagnosis or read the history of treatment that he or she may have undergone, Ganet-Sigel works on formulating a relationship with the individual. When she worked with children who suffered from emotional disturbance at the Reed Zone Mental Health Center, she read a child's chart only after having worked with the individual for at least two or three sessions and having had an opportunity to formulate her own assessment of the child's difficulty based upon their motoric abilities.

In talking with Ganet-Sigel about her theoretical predispositions we learned that that she considers herself to be an eclectic therapist, but as she cautioned,

> . . . electic doesn't mean mish-mash . . . [or] . . . anything you want to do. Instead you need to have a sufficient knowledge base of theories and then determine what theories you might consider blending. However it is equally important that you have a firm understanding of why you would blend particular theories . . . in terms of my own theoretical framework, I would blend psychoanalytical or at least psychodynamic, developmental, (I ascribe to many of Erickson's beliefs), object relations, and humanistic into my approach. With regard to the humanistic theories, I believe that the philosophy of

humanism is crucial to becoming an effective therapist and although I would be hard pressed to select one singular theorist that I ascribe to, I certainly believe in and practice many of the tenets described by Sullivan and Chace.

Chace taught all of her students about Sullivan's interpersonal theory. In terms of the psychodynamic approach, I see myself somewhat affiliated with Freud, but I wander from Freud at certain times. I am not convinced that the id is the only thing that makes you function. I concur with Freud that there is a connection between past experiences and memories and current behavior, but I also believe it is critical to appreciate and understand the client's developmental experiences. Oftentimes, the dance/movement therapy process focuses primarily on developmental issues endemic to experiences incurred while the client was a child, during their pre-teenage age or teenage years. Ultimately dance/movement therapy is about working with the client in the here and now and establishing a therapeutic alliance. The dance/movement therapist must attune himself/herself to the client in order to establish a therapeutic alliance.

My techniques would start with Chacian ideas. Chacian ideas are body actions, rhythms, therapeutic movement relationships, and symbolism. As a therapist, you work with those entities. Working with these ideas during movement helps people change and get in touch with their internal feelings. However I don't use the Chacian techniques exclusively in my practice because the techniques of circle and keeping people safe and within boundaries are used for certain populations that the private practitioner doesn't typically see. I tend to use Chacian techniques in my work with groups because these techniques are embedded in the themes that guide movement. Remember that the techniques that you use really do depend upon what population you are working with. A simple technique involves considering whether you should have your eyes open or closed during warm up. For example, a veteran dance/movement therapist would never have your eyes closed with psychotics because they realize that these clients tend to enter a fantasy world and get lost in outer space. While this is perhaps a minor technique, it would be important information to the novice therapist and it makes a difference.

Overall,. . . I totally believe that in order to change some of the dysfunctional behaviors that people come in with you do have to connect to their roots. Because if you can get connect to the roots and see that they no longer have to produce weeds, they can produce flowers. These ideas offer a working framework from within which you work, but you adjust it and modify it according to the clients' needs. Learning about these and other ideas are an important part of a professional program of study for the aspiring dance/movement therapist.

Another one of the philosophies that I have relates to my work with private clients. Remember, however, that private clients are much different than hospitalized and institutionalized clients. Private clients are people who are in some ways still functioning out there in the world. They can walk into your office on their own two feet and they can leave on time and not have to fall into somebody's arms as with hospitalized patients very often. While hospitalized patients can get through with the dance/movement therapy session, things may still become stirred up inside of them. However within the hospital setting, they have a social worker, a psychiatric nurse, other clients on their wards, that can offer them impromptu support. The intensity of feelings that may become stirred may cause some patients to literally fall in staff's arms. They may need to be held and nurtured so that they can negotiate their pain. On other hand, private clients have to be able to walk out of the office and be able to function on their own. So I am talking right now about the private client.

One of the classical questions that often emerges is: What is the appropriate treatment for this person versus another person? My belief is that everyone who comes to me in private practice, regardless of what they state as their problem, is that they are not coping with that problem well because there is something faulty in their own self-esteem, in their ability to like themselves, or trust themselves. So the therapeutic process with everybody begins to a certain extent by focusing on self-image, body-image, self-esteem, and trust. When clients feel they can trust me, trust themselves, and trust what they are really feeling and begin to like themselves and say, "hey I'm okay, I can handle this," then we begin to work together on their specific issues.

Part of my job is to observe the quality of their movement and their habitual patterns. Even if I sense I have observed a habitual pattern, I never point this out at the beginning. This allows me the time and space to assess what I have seen, and to affirm or refute initial impressions. When I feel that there is trust between the client and myself and the client and the group and there is an openness to hearing the critique, then at certain points I will begin to point out that, "are you aware that every time I ask you to go forward or enter someone's space, you always do it with your hands pushed back or with your arms folded or you enter sideways? Are you aware that you always do that?" This is the beginning of making people aware and then what does that mean? What is the difference if you enter straight forward, halfway or sideways? The answer is that different ways of moving produce different kinds of feelings. For example, if a client moves tentatively to the words push and pull, it might be because he/she is afraid. Thus understanding the quality of movement provides the therapist with information. Observing hesitancy may be the result of fear or repressed traumatic memories that are being held in the upper torso.

Now the kind of observation I am describing should be the hallmark of any effective dance/movement therapist. The difference between my approach and others is that I start working with clients, regardless of what they suggest their issue is, on building self-esteem and establishing trust. I start work with clients at this place because very often I see in my groups and with individuals that these are common issues that influence their adaptive functioning. Now the techniques used may be different for individual clients. Although the techniques used for individual and group clients differ, the focus remains similar. However, I always encourage clients to share what they think their issues are. I communicate to clients that I want to hear their stories and what they are coming in with, and what they feel their problems are.

Ganet-Sigel offers some suggestions for working with clients who suffer from neuroses. The issues that movement is likely to address include: body image, relaxation, separation, sexuality, anger, fears, intimacy, regression, aging, problem solving, self-esteem, trust, focusing. Rather than asking clients to focus on the word "anger," Ganet-Sigel recommends that dance/movement therapists use different movement words and techniques such as (1) music to produce a certain feeling, (2) imagery, (3) developmental stages of childhood, (4) transitional objects, (5) free association in movement, (6) dreams, and (7) roles that facilitate the client's expression of emotions. Therapists are advised to be flexible and use fewer words to control the client. Sometimes the powerfulness of movement evokes a charged response from the client in which he/she becomes enraged, for example, and acts out. In this situation, the therapist should ask the client to share what they believe really happened and to describe what they wish would happen or their fantasy of what should happen.

Ganet-Sigel's Group Dance/Movement Therapy Techniques

Clients who suffer somatic tension from repressed feelings can also be helped in group dance/movement therapy. In this context they can learn how they are perceived by others and how their behaviors perpetuate unsatisfactory relationships (Stanton, 1991). However clients must be able to, or learn, to trust one another, and delay or alter ". . . their own gratification in service to other group members as well as the capacity to receive and do direct individual work in the presence of others" (Lewis, 1986, p. 201). The client's movement experiences may be facilitated through the use of images or themes to bring about experimenting with different kinds of movement, encouraging self-directed forms of movement exploration, moving in synchronicity with the client, or verbalization in response to movement. Therapeutic change occurs through an interplay of group experiences and what Yalom (1975) has identified as curative factors. These factors: universality, altruism, the development of socializing techniques, imitative behavior, interpersonal learning, corrective recapitulation of the primary family group, catharsis, group cohesiveness, existential factors, the instillation of hope and imparting new knowledge, highlight the valuable use of dance/movement therapy. A process that progresses from movement through association with images to interpretation occurs as group members begin to the see the relationship between movements, images, and feelings (Stanton, 1991).

Group therapy offers an environment for clients to experience positive object relations and promotes a sense of belongingness to the group. Rhythmic activity is one of many factors that can stimulate feelings of unity and solidarity (Thomson, 1997). Repressed memories that are enacted during movement can be shared by others, rather than judged and criticized. Group members' acceptance and support of one another offers a safe environment for clients to reveal their innermost pain, strengthen their egos, and work towards adaptive coping.

What techniques does Ganet-Sigel use in her group therapy work with clients? Among the techniques she has used are: (1) mirroring, (2) working in triads, (3) the progressive development of primary movements, (4) moving to specific words such as *swing, stretch, bounce, push, dodge, bend, twist, shake, pull, strike,* among others (5) moving to specific words with a partner, where one individual has been assigned the role of a parent, (6) doing the same as the previous step, where the other partner changes roles and becomes the parent, (7) sculpting others in triads and dyads, and (8) witnessing the sculpturing of others in triads and dyads among others.

Groups are comprised by three stages: (1) warm-up activities, (2) the development of a theme, and (3) closure activities. The purpose of the warm-up activities are (1) to relax the group and observe what is coming up for and being released by clients from which the therapist is then able to assist in choosing a theme, (2) to provide a common movement pattern for all, and (3) to provide a "blank canvas" upon which the patients might begin to pair movement with emotional expression of themselves. During warm-up activities the therapist observes and reflects the dynamics which clients start to superimpose (Lewis, 1986). During the second stage, development of the theme, ". . . [therapists] are to pick up planning and enlarge upon existing patterns which manifest themselves . . ." (Lewis, 1986, p. 201). However, group sessions remain loosely structured to allow thematic material that is revealed during client movement to further exploration. During the third stage, the closure activities, the therapist (1) insures that clients regain their individual control mechanisms and (2) facilitates individual cognitive awareness of what has occurred during movement and helps clients come to understand how their movement relates to their emotions.

> Conscious awareness via verbal associations, insight producing interpretations, and/or comments by the therapist and client/patient are made pertaining to the relationship of the unconscious material to the individual's experience of present life and the development of further consciousness (Lewis, 1986, p. 284).

Jane uses a variety of techniques to guide the group movement process. Table 1.2 below provides an overview of techniques that she uses during warm-up activities and during the development of a theme (using transitional objects, moving to specific words, moving specific body parts, mirroring (shadowing) and free association (movement).

Table 1.2 GANET-SIGEL'S COMPENDIUM OF MOVEMENT TECHNIQUES FOR GROUP THERAPY

Warm-up activities techniques

Circle warm-up
self warm-up (15 minutes)
massage warm-up
guided warm-up

Techniques to use during the development of a theme

Moving with transitional objects
ropes—stretch cloth, puff ball–bonding rope
transitional objects (balloons, scarves, ropes, stretch ropes, stretch cloth)

Moving to specific words[2]
10 movement words (stretch, swing, pull, push, bend, twist, dodge, strike, shake, bounce)
walk, run, skip, hop, gallop, leap, high, low, large, small, fast, slow, circle, diagonal, forward, back
weak—light, heavy
close—far, toward
away—hello, good-bye
yes, no, I won't, I will—I can, I can't, I should
open close
feminine masculine
child—adult
sustain, fragment
play, joy, under, above
give & take, down, under, over

Moving specific body parts
move with separate body parts leading:

the part I like best	dislike most
hardest to move	easiest to move
emotionally stressful	emotionally joyful
others like	others dislike

Mirroring (shadowing)
draw self—move self
draw tree—move tree
mirror a partner's movements

Free association (movement)

with music	against music
right side	left side

---

[2] This is not an exhaustive list because Ganet-Sigel often selects new words during the process of therapy.

**Table 1.2 GANET-SIGEL'S COMPENDIUM OF MOVEMENT
TECHNIQUES FOR GROUP THERAPY (continued)**

Additional words and techniques[3]

past, present, future

termination

dyads—triads

statues

entering space

roles

names

colors

favorite toys

birth to present

other potent words

parental roles (nurturing, rejecting, teasing, possessive, controlling, permissive, playful)

elements (clouds, stars, sun, moon, water, fire, earth, wind)

flowers

animals

colors

sheets (womb)

focus—trongrelate

only with facial expressions

negative and positive sides

regression

trust (blindfold—dyads)

symbolic objects (3) make choices

parachute

batakas—anger

Theory into Practice

In the following section Ganet-Sigel describes her work with a very ill young woman, Sylvia[4] (see Chapter 6). Next, the psychiatrist, Dr. Russet[5], who referred the woman to Ganet-Sigel, discusses his perspective about the role that dance/movement therapy placed in her recovery.

> Sylvia entered therapy as a very regressed individual. I worked with her almost from her birth. For months and months we sat together and all I did was hold and rock her in my arms. Essentially the therapy consisted primarily of what object relations theorists refer to as bonding. I worked with Sylvia to re-bond with her, a process that a healthy parent typically provides for his/her children.

---

[3] These are additional words and techniques that can be used wherever the therapist and the client find them useful. This is list is not exhaustive.

[4] Sylvia is a pseudonym. The real name of the patient is not used here.

[5] Dr. Russet is a pseudonym. The real name of the psychiatrist is not used here.

Therapy focused on re-bonding and trying to eliminate and eradicate the abuse and traumas that Sylvia had experienced in her early childhood and to replace an absence of symbiosis. The object relations theorists have pointed out that the individual has to become symbiotic before separation can take place. Concurring with objects relations theorists about the importance of bonding, Ganet-Sigel related that:

> . . . Working with the severely regressed client who has been abused requires that the therapist assume the role of the surrogate parent so that the client has an opportunity to re-bond. This technique permits the client to re-establish their kinesthetic system and visceral knowledge. They may need to help the client regress developmentally to the phase where he/she became arrested and be born at the re-bonding. In Sylvia's case, she needed the therapist to facilitate this regression and healthy re-bonding so that she could individuate.

> The technique for Sylvia was totally different than what I would have used for other individuals or groups. In her case, there was so much abuse. What is important to realize about her case is that she was totally disconnected from her body and mind to such a degree that she didn't even know that she had a self. Therefore her treatment had to start actually from birth. I had to start as her mother, since she needed so much caring and nurturing. The only way I could nurture her was to put her in my arms and rock her.

> Initially therapy focused on bonding with Sylvia as mother and child by giving her what most babies hopefully receive is wonderful touching and nurturing. The type of touching and nurturing I am describing facilitates infants' ability to feel their bodies and realize that they are loved. That is one of the foundations of developing a healthy mother-child bond. Within the context of this relationship is where infants can experience trust.

> So it was at this developmental point in time that I began intervening with Sylvia. Other people don't have to go that far back. For others who need to develop a better understanding of themselves, I would use guided warm-ups to help them get in touch with their viscera, move while looking at themselves in the mirror, encourage the expansion of various movement patterns, and eventually point to changes in their movement patterns that I had observed over a period of time.

Although Sylvia is healing, reportedly she still has trouble negotiating change. Ganet-Sigel explains why Sylvia may be experiencing this type of difficulty.

> Even though the client experiences healing, there is residue. Sylvia was in a lot pain and overcame lots of obstacles. There are levels of how we respond to certain things. Sylvia responded a

little bit more actively, while for other people these responses may not be as stressful. Making changes requires shifting. People who experience dance therapy or any kind of body therapy where they are made to be aware of what's going inside, become more attuned to their internal, visceral, kinesthetic responses. Because of their emergent awareness of what is happening to them, they are sometimes more uncomfortable than people who have never allowed themselves to become aware. There are times in my own life when I say to myself why am I so aware of every trickle, bubble, wrinkle, burp, and gas and tiny little pain coming across . . . at times I find it disconcerting to be so acutely aware, however then of course I start thinking of what is it connected to. Sometimes we can go overboard instead of realizing that we are just experiencing being a normal response to normal bodily functioning.

Sylvia was experiencing intense difficulty due to a combination of issues. She was going in and out of psychosis with no relief and was not amenable to medicinal intervention. Verbal therapy was also limited for her. The psychiatrist believed that dance/movement therapy might offer her a chance to experience some relief from her symptoms. According to Dr. Russet:

> Sylvia would experience an uncomfortableness and an anger oftentimes in different situations and relationships, even just thinking about things, such as thinking about her Father or Mother. That would result in her feeling and experiencing a lot of turbulent emotions, turbulent feelings, and turbulent physical experiences inside of herself. So what the dance/movement therapy did was . . . it connected with those feelings and experiences.

Dr. Russet suggested that Ganet-Sigel's form of treatment was much more effective in treating the things that confronted Sylvia. He began to realize how beneficial dance/movement therapy was.

> After I determined that the movement had made such an impact on things [for Sylvia], and that it was just so helpful, [I realized] that was something that I wasn't able to provide or do. As a result of the changes I observed in Sylvia's behavior, I began to refer people who I thought had difficulty working on their feelings through talking on a regular basis to Ganet-Sigel.
>
> The way I conceptualized things was that dance/movement therapy directly connected with the person's innermost experience and feelings. The process was able to impact on clients by facilitating a deep physical connection which was not accessible oftentimes through talking or listening.

The reason that dance/movement was effective with Sylvia according to Dr. Russet was the movement process itself.

That was what worked in my opinion. That was the difference between Jane's dance/movement therapy and other people's psychotherapy. It was the physical nature of the dance/movement therapy that made a difference.

Commenting about his perceptions of dance/movement therapy, Dr. Russet revealed that:

I haven't formally studied it so I just tell you my limited knowledge and understanding of it. Through the movement, the person, the client, the patient is able to connect with their innermost and deepest feelings, emotions, and experiences and through Jane's therapeutic understanding, she can help the person change those innermost and deepest feelings, emotions, and experience in a therapeutic way. There's a physical connection through the movement therapy to the person's experiences, somatic experiences and emotional experiences. And through that physical connection, the person's emotions and somatic experiences can actually be changed.

How did the therapeutic process impact Sylvia's well-being? Did the therapy help bring material to a consciousness level and help her realize that she had a choice about how she reacted? Did therapy help Sylvia learn how to replace rageful behavior with more adaptive coping mechanisms? Russet suggested that Sylvia's experiences were not consciously-mediated, and that in fact, the dance/movement therapy processes were complementary to the type of illness which from she suffered.

. . . it wasn't a matter of thinking, choosing or anything intellectual. The way I saw it that it directly connected to it physically and impacted it physically and it wasn't a matter of thinking or choice, it was a whole re-patterning of physical experience. I really saw it as a physical process and not an intellectual process, in the physiological, immunological sense.

Not knowing if dance/movement therapy would be effective for Sylvia, Dr. Russet confessed that it really was an experiment. However, seeing how Sylvia had changed, his openness and acceptance of dance/movement therapy grew even more. He shared:

[I] had no experience with it whatsoever before that and I just happened to be in the right place at the right time just as Sylvia was in the right place at the right time. I had no knowledge of [dance/movement therapy] previously.

I just experienced Jane as very strong and brave and she had the ability to . . . I call it "shifting energy." She had the ability to move a person's center . . . She has the ability to connect and then help the person move . . .

Establishing Therapeutic Relationships

What steps does a dance/movement therapist take in establishing a relationship (alliance) and in initiating treatment with private practice clients? What is a therapeutic alliance? Lewis suggested that is the moment

> . . . when client and teacher recognize and accept the client's beginning attitude, *without judging it.* The cue is taken from [the therapist]; the client is waiting to see [the therapist's] reactions. . . . What is wanted is a genuine involvement; it is only from the involvement that the process itself can begin. . . . (Lewis, 1986, p. 74).

The therapeutic alliance is crucial to the success of the therapist-patient relationship.

The following diagram (see Figure 1.1) illustrates a process model of the development of a therapeutic alliance with private practice clients. Note that the therapist uses material that is revealed by clients to guide them in making adaptive behavioral changes and coping mechanisms.

Figure 1.1   A process model for establishing therapeutic relationships

1. Assess the client's movement repertoire.

2. Establish treatment goals (which often change during the course of therapy).

3. Select movement themes.

4. Initiate the process of movement.

5. Use movement to facilitate behavioral change. (This will facilitate bringing movement patterns to conscious awareness.)

6. Help client understand how observed movement patterns relate to current behavior.

7. Help client identify how to change dysfunctional movement patterns and replace them with more healthy coping mechanisms.

Conclusion

Ganet-Sigel's orientation to therapy is considered eclectic, having evolved from a mixture of Freudian psychology, developmental psychology, and object-relations theory. While she accepts Freud's views that the client's environment and background are contextually important to child development, she rejects the notion that the libido is inextricably linked to all childhood traumas and conflicts. She views Freudian and developmental psychology as closely linked and important to guiding the therapist's interpretation. However, she perceives object-relations as a more critical facet to analyzing clients' issues.

There's a strong connection between the mind and body; however, often we may focus so much on the mind that the body becomes neglected. In dance movement therapy, the body is awakened. The body is going to tell on you. While an individual may say one thing, the body's movement might be demonstrating a totally different story. Someone may be moving a certain way and thinking they're presenting themselves a certain way, and yet the body may moving in an entirely different way. In therapy, clients begin to listen to their bodies and the dialogue inside. Dance/movement therapy promotes our ability listen to ourselves and to notice what the body is telling others.

Engaging in dance/movement therapy is a journey. Sometimes depending on the presenting issues, clients may experience their own private journey through hell, and while feeling pain and discomfort is destabilizing, these experiences may precede clients' realization that they can chose more adaptive forms of coping. As clients learn about their own particular patterns of responding, they also learn that there are healthier ways of functioning. It is important to recognize that dance/movement therapy is not art or indulgent self-expression. The therapeutic aim is to effect a change in the client's behavior. In this light, the process of dance/movement therapy shares a common purpose with cognitive-behavioral therapy. As clients become more in touch with their somatic experiences, they are likely to engage more frequently in self-talk as they work towards experimenting with the expression of more adaptive behaviors.

In dance/movement therapy clients discover different options and have an opportunity to experience different ways of responding and exploring feelings that may have been evoked. As with any form of therapy, including dance/movement, clients may experience regression, but the combination of kinesthetic and verbal aspects of the process tend to encourage self-discovery and progress rather than stasis.

CHAPTER 2

The Dance/Movement Therapist as Pioneer and Program Developer

Guiding Questions

1. *Why is it important for the dance/movement therapist to have training in dance?*
2. *What are the major movements in the emergence of dance/movement therapy in the Midwest?*
3. *What can the dance/movement therapist who is interested in program development learn from Ganet-Sigel's pioneering?*
4. *What are some of the characteristics that are essential to becoming an effective therapist?*
5. *In what ways has Ganet-Sigel influenced her students, as well as colleagues in dance/movement therapy and allied fields?*

What is usually referred to as intuition, even granting some innate ability, is the result of many years of learning and appreciating human and family processes (Satir and Baldwin, 1983, p. 225). Essentially, the therapist must be willing to live with the ambiguity of a very dynamic system, in a constant state of flux, with many variables apt to erupt at any time (Satir and Baldwin, 1983, p. 229).

In this chapter the authors describe Ganet-Sigel's career development. In the first two sections that describe her early and latter career, they provide an overview of her contributions to the field of dance/movement therapy. To help the reader understand the woman who became a national leader in her field, they address the question, What can be learned from the work of a pioneer and program developer? They also describe her role in helping to bring dance/movement therapy to the Midwest and Chicago. Next, the authors address the questions: What are the characteristics of a dance/movement therapist? Who is Jane Ganet-Sigel as a person and a woman? To offer the reader an impression of Ganet-Sigel as an individual, they describe how students, clients, colleagues, friends, and family regard her.

Ganet-Sigel's Early Career

Brief chronological overview Before entering the field of dance/
movement therapy, Ganet-Sigel was a dance and drama instructor.
After attending the University of Illinois from 1944–1946 as a dance
major, she married and raised four children. While experiencing major
changes in her own life, a divorce from her first husband and still raising two of her sons, she began attending Northeastern Illinois University. She became a certified social worker (CSW) in 1968 and
completed a Bachelor of Science degree in psychology (1972). Also
during this time period, in 1972, she became both a registered
dance/movement therapist (DTR) and certified activity therapist. Subsequently she began graduate studies at Governor's State University and
was awarded a Master of Arts degree in human development in 1973.
She earned her association of registered dance/movement therapist
(ADTR) status in 1982. From 1978–1982, she directed the Bachelor of
Arts program in dance/movement therapy at Columbia College and
taught the Introduction to Dance/Movement Therapy course until
1983 at DePaul University. She also served as guest faculty at the Institute for Therapy Through the Arts from 1976 to 1985. In 1976, she was
a field faculty member in the school of social work at the University of
Illinois in Chicago. From 1967 to 1977, she worked as a dance therapist
and group therapist at the Chicago Reed Mental Health Center Therapeutic Nursery School. From 1964 to 1977 she was a consultant to
school districts and the juvenile protective association. She also worked
as a dance/movement therapist and group therapist with disturbed
youth and adults in psychiatric hospitals, mental health centers, and
halfway houses. Additionally she supervised almost all of the aspiring
dance/movement therapists in Chicago and the surrounding area from
the late 1960's to the mid-1980's. Prior to this, from 1947–1964, she
held many positions in dance and drama. She was the Director of the
Dance Department for the Bernard Horwich Community Center in
Chicago (1960–1964), the Director and Owner of the Creative Workshop in Skokie, IL (1954–1959), the Program Director of the Children's
Program for the Jewish People's Institute (1947–1950) as well as
dance/drama specialist at the same agency (1946–1947). She also grad-
uated from the Actors' Company of Chicago in 1947.

Detailed chronology Intuitively, Ganet-Sigel always believed there
was something positive about dance; even as young as 2½, she recalls
that ". . . dance was therapy for me." Beginning from the time she was
a young girl enrolled in ballet and modern dance classes and continu-
ing into her professional role as a dance and drama instructor, Ganet-
Sigel witnessed and experienced a positive energy that emerged during
dance. Although parental disapproval steered her away from seeking a
career as a professional performer her feelings about the positive power
of dance became reified during the time she taught dance and drama to
young children.

Remembering Ganet-Sigel as a little girl and her love for dance, one of her cousins shared:

> . . . when Jane Ann and her family moved back to Chicago, I saw a lot of her. She was always such a cute little curly-headed girl. Jane Ann was always dancing, too. One summer day while I was studying dancing with a man named Fran Scanlon downtown in the Lyon and Healy building, I went with Jane Ann and her mother to her dance. [At that time Jane Ann was attending] a neighborhood dance school. When I got home, I told her mother I thought she was wasting her money with that teacher. And if she could see her way clear to take Jane Ann downtown to Fran's, I thought he would do something with her. So sure enough, her mother did, and her career today is part of the result of that, I'm sure.

As a young woman, Ganet-Sigel often found herself wondering about the relationship between dance and the changes in behavior that she had experienced and observed among her students. During her own reflection, one question seemed to occur repeatedly. Why do people seem to feel better about themselves when they are dancing? Then, one day in 1964, she read about the work of Marian Chace, the woman credited for developing dance/movement therapy. To her amazement, not only was this inductive relationship creditable, in fact an entire discipline had been devoted to understanding how dance affected emotion and how emotion affected behavior. She realized that properly implemented, dance techniques could be used to help others experience healing. At that point she felt absolutely convinced that the idea of using dance to help people emotionally was just what she had observed in her work with young children. During presentations and workshops, Ganet-Sigel has often shared with her audiences that:

> I knew that there was something about movement and emotion . . . I used to get letters from parents of my students that would say something like, I don't know how good a dancer my child is because of your class, but there is a humanism in her due to it.

Ganet-Sigel wrote Marian Chace and was accepted into her course. After taking a two-week dance/movement therapy course from Chace in 1966 at the Turtle Bay Music School in New York, she became one of 73 charter members of the newly formed American Dance/Movement Therapy Association (ADTA). Although her family was puzzled by her intense need to do this, she went to New York and "in some way felt that this course viscerally and kinetically was something I had been doing all my life."

> Voila, I came back to Chicago, knew my goals in life and suddenly, I was a dance therapist, but I also knew I needed to learn a new vocabulary, was functioning in a vacuum and had no one to talk to about this. I did keep in touch with Marian Chace and she

wrote a letter to Dr. Dyrud at University of Chicago telling him
to keep in touch with me.

Along with the other members, but alone in the Midwest, she learned
the theories, techniques, and ethics of the field by staying in touch with
the people in the East and observing others. Chace's course motivated
her to return to school and look for work in her new field.
"I proceeded to go back to school to get my psychology and human
development degrees, and when the ADTA was chartered on October
29, 1966, I became one of the 73 chartered members."

> Being alone here made things difficult. People were scattered
> around the Midwest, continuity and sameness was complicated
> by our distance from one another. I had to draw from my inner
> sensations to develop a trust for this therapy and believe that there
> *was* a meaning.

However, even as Ganet-Sigel undertook career changes, she recalls the
conflict she experienced. "I continued to struggle for years between
dancing professionally, doing soap opera on radio, going back to school
to be a social worker or staying home and being mother of the year with
my children."

Later on in 1967, Ganet-Sigel contacted Evelyn Baumann, a psychiatric social worker at the Reed Mental Health Center, and successfully sold herself as a dance-movement therapist. The day center
treatment program offered services for young children with severe emotional disturbances. Often the children suffered from profound functional retardation or neurological impairment or both in addition to
emotional disturbances. The objective was to provide early intervention to young children and prevent future hospitalization while maintaining them within their own families and communities, to avoid the
dislocation and fragmentation of care that institutionalization causes.
The work also involved intensive intervention with families. The program was created by Illinois Department of Mental Health within a
new facility known as the Chicago-Reed Mental Health Center and
part of a state hospital where in the past such children would be institutionalized. Children aged two to six were accepted for treatment.
Their combined diagnoses included autism, psychosis, anaclitic depression, character disorder, and severe delayed ego development. The children were frequently profoundly functionally retarded, neurologically
impaired or both. Typically they attended school five days a week, from
9 a.m.–1 p.m. along flexible scheduling that was implemented dependent upon each child's needs (Baumann, 1976).

The program combined specialized psycho-educational techniques
with corrective socialization experiences. Classes primarily emphasized
emotional growth, but fostering academic gains were also an integral
part of the children's experiences. As children progressed to sufficient
levels of adaptive functioning they were gradually placed back into public or parochial school settings (Metronews, 1973). Specialists in a variety of fields were hired to provide a multi-team therapeutic involvement.

The classroom concept was utilized with an early childhood specialist as the "teacher therapist" with two teacher assistants and approximately five children in a group. This meant that it was possible for teachers to relate to specific children. The support staff included social workers for the families, speech pathologists, and child psychologists. Children with severe emotional disorders including autism attended the school. Referrals frequently came from hospital staff who were involved with the families of hospitalized parents and were aware of the special needs of others still at home.

Baumann hired Ganet-Sigel, and she began her career by working with severely emotionally disturbed children at the center's therapeutic day school. Describing her work Baumann remarked that:

> . . . she did more than just dance therapy, . . . she had a way of relating to a child, and . . . used the dance therapy as a human being related. She would come into the room, get involved with the children, especially ones who particularly at that time needed her. [She] is more than just a person who gets involved with movement and dance. She's a therapist, and as a therapist, she is able to . . . develop empathy with a child. We had some children who couldn't talk, and . . . dance therapy [offered] one way of reaching a child who you couldn't reach any other way. The child could feel Jane's presence and could relate to Jane in a way that otherwise they couldn't communicate verbally.

One of her colleagues, a psychiatrist, shared some observations about her work.

> What I remember most was how intrigued and impressed I was with Jane's work with the children. These were very young, mostly I would say maybe two-and-a-half or three- to five-year-old children all seriously developmentally delayed in one or more ways, all very challenging in terms of resistance to therapy. It was a wonderful school with teachers who were essentially the therapists. They were nursery school teachers, but because of the nature of the children they had to be therapists, so what they were doing nowadays would be called educational therapy. Jane and I were part of the team. I was a psychiatric consultant, and I'd come once a week, and we would have staffings and we would meet to talk about development and we would focus on maybe one child every week.
>
> Jane would work with all of the children; that was impressive. I think I was able to observe her work and I can't remember a single child who was not engaged in the work with Jane. Most impressive to me was her work with the children who were withdrawn and unreachable to all other people on the staff. But Jane had a way of using her techniques and herself to engage children who were in their own worlds and she would imitate the child and the child would be intrigued to be affirmed in such a nonthreatening way. The child would then imitate back in such a way a movement language would be established. It was quite wonderful to see. To me it was entirely new.

> Being a psychiatrist, I was a talker, and I got nowhere with
> these children. But Jane knew that language through motion
> would reach them. I really was astounded that withdrawn chil-
> dren could be enticed into human contact through Jane's work.
> That's what stands out to me in my memory of those times.

During the 1960's, Ganet-Sigel was the only registered
dance/movement therapist in the Midwest, although few people understood or appreciated what dance/movement was. While perhaps not
unexpected, she found severe resistance as she tried to introduce the
conceptual nature of her work to medicinally trained therapists.

> I, alone in Chicago, was struggling with finishing my degree,
> dancing and raising my growing family. I kept selling myself as a
> dance therapist, expanding the philosophy of body and mind
> integration. No one knew what I was talking about, nor did I
> completely, but that didn't stop me. I must admit, the less I knew,
> the more outraged I was when people looked at me strangely
> when I went to offer my services at a psychiatric hospital.

Ganet-Sigel recalls the less than tepid response of the hospital director
who asked if she wanted him to do the cha-cha. Although she stalked
out of the room, today she jokingly admits that she would have replied
"Yes," and used movement to draw him out if the same scenario was to
repeat itself. Ganet-Sigel endured a lot of door slamming because the
Chicago medical community was not receptive to a form of psychotherapy predicated upon the assumption that the mind and body
were integrated and that used dance to facilitate therapeutic healing.

> During this same period — I was going around to all kinds of
> facilities and offering my services. It was here that I developed
> techniques, ideas, learned to work with catatonics, elderly, adoles-
> cents, schizophrenics, and others. I had free reign to do what I
> wanted to do.
> I was member at large on the National Board at that time, [and]
> was asked to host the 1968 National Conference. Mildred Dickin-
> son and I were the only 2 in Chicago, can you imagine now, plan-
> ning a national conference, all alone! Well, we took the challenge.
> We worked hard and long, but that was the year of the national
> political convention in Chicago, and the riots and then Major
> Daley did not compliment our city too well. National voted to
> take the conference out of Chicago several months prior to the
> conference date. Needless to say, I was devastated, having spent so
> much time in preparing for the conference. Instead the 3rd Annu-
> al Conference October 25–27, 1968 came to Madison. Although
> I worked along with others on the arrangements for the conference
> it was with bitterness and anger. A highlight of this conference was
> Marian Chace, Jarl E. Dyrud and Jean Erdman, who talked about
> the meaning of movement as human expression and as an artistic
> communication.

During the time I was completing my master's degree, I had a wonderful mentor who encouraged me to teach a course in dance/movement therapy. This endeavor actually resulted in the development of several courses, Introduction to Dance Therapy, a course in dance/music/art for children with emotional disturbances and many workshops for staffs at different homes for the retarded, psychotic and disturbed children. Those of us in the Midwest were so busy, trying to find work or making people aware of dance therapy, that most of the time our only contact was at annual meetings. That's where we brought our ideas together on theories and techniques. Throughout this time I had a distinct feeling of isolation and then suddenly, Marian Chace died!

Problems begin to arise with the individuals who were isolated in situations in the midwest. The harnessing and taming came in with the inception of the registry in 1972. Guidelines for beginning DTR were set, many people not only in Midwest but in other isolated parts of the country, found it difficult to abide by everything. Many were made to feel inferior or inadequate simply because of the struggle just to do dance therapy, let alone get supervision from newly existing DTR scattered in the Midwest. At this time the Midwest included Ohio, Michigan, Indiana, Illinois, Wisconsin, Kansas, Missouri, Iowa, Nebraska, Minnesota, North and South Dakota, Colorado, Texas, Arkansas, Louisiana, and Oklahoma. Talk about knowing your boundaries! Anyplace that didn't fit into the West Coast or East Coast was Midwest. The 8th annual conference was held in Kansas City, in 1973.

I personally was reaching out everywhere in Chicago. A demonstration at Highland Park High School for Creative Arts Week, Jan Isaac-Henry now (chairman of ethics committee of ADTA) heard me speak about dance therapy and has often told me this talk motivated her into becoming a dance therapist. While doing workshops throughout Illinois and the Midwest, I also started introductory classes at Columbia College Chicago in 1974. Meanwhile I taught courses for a mental health certification and served as field faculty for several colleges. I gave workshops, seminars, and training throughout the city, since I was the only DTR in town.

The first newsletter that brought people together in the Midwest helped many of us realize that we shared some common concerns. One issue was related to receiving supervision from existing DTR. As a result of this dilemma many of the Midwestern dance/movement therapists had difficulty successfully completing the requirements for licensing. In April of 1976 I played a co-leadership role in organizing the first Midwest dance/movement therapy conference. Dr. Dyrud spoke at that conference. And we had over 100 people from all over the Midwest. At the national conference in DC that fall, thirty enthusiastic Midwest members met and began procedures for becoming a chapter. In 1979 — there were 5 approved graduate degree programs in dance therapy, none in the Midwest. In 1979 Minneapolis hosted the Midwest conference, 1980 in Indianapolis and by 1982 we began to feel even more scattered and too big an area. Many area therapists worked hard to develop identities as dance/movement therapists, challenging current ethics, policies and guidelines. However our efforts to keep our heads above water as therapists became overwhelming. Many of us experienced a sense of isolation due to a lack of supervision, frustration in meeting requirements for registration, lack of professional support, difficulty finding jobs, and the absence of a Midwest newsletter. The question of getting registered through an alternate route degree continued to be a heavy issue.

Meanwhile I organized the Chicago Collective, almost insisting that students and professionals come together regularly in order to be on top of all the issues both nationally and regionally. Our Midwest attempted to meet in clusters, putting the Midwest in 3 clusters instead of all together. Each cluster met independently and began to address the issues of their particular regions. Responses to mailed questionnaires helped determine the future of our chapters and regions. In 1982 — my proposal for a M.A. in Dance/Movement Therapy was accepted by Columbia College Chicago. Twelve students entered the first class. In 1986 the program had more than 30 students. Today our program has 45–50 students each semester. Of course, in order to attain accreditation, dance/movement therapy programs had to demonstrate having met ADTA's guidelines for approved programs, training, administration, and program development that helped students fulfill requirements for a two standard registry.

"Coming of Age" was the theme for the National Conference in November, 1986. Chicago came through in a pinch when Texas withdrew from chairing the conference. Chicago took it on, not minding hard work involved. Many area dance/movement therapists volunteered to help put the conference together. By 1986 Chicago now had 6 ADTR's capable of doing supervision and private practice, who were engaged in raising the consciousness in the Midwest of allied professionals and others regarding our professional identity. Additionally 45 hospitals were willing to accept field placements and internships as a result of my constant public relations campaign, speeches, in-services, and communication. Today we have over 100 internship sites.

During my career I've done radio talk shows, TV shows and have spoken at psychiatric meetings. While there are many stories I have left out, I believe I had offered an overview of the history of the development of dance/movement therapy in the Midwest. This process has been challenging at times, especially when ADTA did not recognized the midwest contingent's search for meaning, when they've had panels and evenings of nostalgia about the stages of growth of the "family" or organization, when the late bloomers, the midwesterners, have been ignored, even though the Midwest had been acquiring the strengths to transcend and take chances in each new stage of development.

> Sometimes the struggle seemed overwhelming. However I am convinced that those who succeed in their anticipated adult world thereby shoulder the obligation of forwarding the future of dance/movement therapy. I have loved my work and believe that it has been worth the struggle to attain identity, find alternative ways to earn licensing, locate jobs, and develop training programs.

Several of her former students, now colleagues, shared their views about Ganet-Sigel's struggle to introduce dance/movement therapy as a credible therapeutic intervention.

> . . . there was resistance everywhere, in the medical community, in academia, even with clients. When I think of Jane having . . . the conviction to struggle against that for all these years, it's a real test of your personal self-esteem as well as your conviction for the work, that dance therapists are sort of testing that at every day. And [I] have an appreciation for that and what that does to a person. It creates vociferousness. [It] makes me appreciate all the more the burden that she's had all these years and that the vociferousness, I believe, that . . . really came out of her determination that dance therapy was going to be an accepted field . . . a respected one.
>
> [She] fought to give life to dance/movement therapy in the Midwest, while developing her own life and private practice. [This] exemplifies one's ability to make contributions to world/personal life simultaneously [and is] an extraordinary example of conviction and actualization.
>
> [Jane is] truly a pioneer in the field of what integrating the body is all about.

However Ganet-Sigel was also recognized by others outside of dance/movement therapy (see Appendix A). In acknowledgement of her contributions to the field, Mayor Harold Washington of Chicago proclaimed that

> ". . . November 5–9, 1986 to be "COMING OF AGE" — JANE GANET-SIGEL DAY IN CHICAGO in recognition of the 21st Annual Conference "Coming of Age" and for the many contributions of Chicagoans and Midwestern Dance Therapists, such as Jane Ganet-Sigel, for devotion to development and growth in this field.

In spite of responses for this new therapeutic modality that ranged from blatant rejection to cynicism, she persevered and was able to get her foot in the door at hospitals, schools, and social service agencies. Single-handedly, she broke down barriers to the field and made a lot of presentations to allied health professionals. She started seeing patients in private practice in 1973 and offered individual and group therapy. The next year, she was asked to teach undergraduate dance/movement therapy courses and direct the Bachelor of Arts program in dance/movement therapy at Columbia College, a position she held until 1982. Then during the same year, at the age of 56, she became the founder and director of one of the five accredited programs in the nation, the Graduate Program of Dance/Movement Therapy at Columbia College Chicago.

In 1974 Ganet-Sigel met Mildred (Millie) Chapin, a renowned art therapist. Together they persevered as a team, acting as saleswomen for art therapy and dance/movement therapy respectively. Chapin described how they met and came to work together.

When I first came to Chicago, I didn't know anyone. I think it was in 1974. I was eager to make contacts in the world of art therapy. Somebody suggested that I see Jane, who was a dance therapist. And the recommendation was that she was wonderful with children, just wonderful, and that we would get along and she could sort of tell me what was going on in Chicago. So I went to meet her . . .

This was well before she started the program at Columbia College . . . but when I met her, that was a dream. . . . She was a working therapist. So our first relationship was one working therapist to another. In different cities. I was coming from Washington, D.C. So I was looking for work opportunities and connections.

. . . our first meeting was about our ways of working with children. And she described her work which was very understandable to me. I told her, of course, that I had been involved in dance for most of my life and had actually been a friend of Marian Chace who began dance therapy . . . a very dear friend of mine in Washington. And together we started the Modern Dance Council in Washington. And I worked with her a little bit at the hospital where she worked. She actually wanted me to be one of her protégés. That was before she set up any kind of teaching operation.

. . . And when [Jane] described her work with children, the physical work, the movement, this was very, very understandable to me. And I could see that she was a person [who] approached the whole idea of therapy in a way that was similar to mine.

It was clear to me that she fully appreciated the sensory, the physical aspects of a human being coming in contact with the world at the very beginning and that this experience was the groundwork for healthy development thereafter. And that people who had problems may not have had problems that far back but that in every way, whether their problems were situated in later stages of life like early childhood, or adolescence, and so on, everyone has the experience of the sensory connection to the world and that through that, through the sensory connection, you can reach people. And they can dialogue with you.

So at our first meeting we had a common understanding of this kind of encounter with the client, not necessarily based on talking or intellectual stuff, or professing this or that or expressing or sharing. It was based on something much more primitive. By primitive, I mean the earliest stages of sensory experience. And that means moving. Moving and touching and smelling and hearing and all that. So, as I say, we didn't have long theoretical discussions in the beginning, but I sensed this and knew it. I was teaching, and so I always had to translate my experience into theory, as I'm doing for you right now. And I understood all of this theoretically as well. But that wasn't the way we talked to each other, necessarily. We sort of understood it.

. . . from the very beginning, [we] appreciated each other, and that developed into something much, much more of friendship as well as professional collegiality. So she gave me some names of people to see. I started teaching in Chicago [and] telling her about the art therapy programs where I'd been teaching at George Washington University in Washington, D.C. So I was very familiar with how to set up a program in universities. I was among the first faculty. I mean, I think the second year of operation or the third, something like that.

So I started working there and was in touch then with a world of expressive therapists working in institutions like hospitals. So we decided at one point that there were a lot of people who wanted to learn about dance therapy; however, there was no program.

[We] decided that this might be a good time to have a course on our own—of course, I was teaching on my own and I think she was, too. We wanted to have this profit from each other's classes. She would teach dance therapy for a certain number of weeks and I would teach art therapy to a different group for a certain number of weeks, and then our group would shift and my group would go to work with her for one or two sessions and vice versa, which was, I thought, a great idea. She did, too.

And so we worked together [and] did the whole thing . . . wrote the brochures, . . . licked stamps and sent them all out and gathered together names . . . it was a big job for the first time to make a mailing list. I mean, we went through the Yellow Pages. I didn't know anybody and she, of course, did but—not everybody . . . we gathered together all the psychologists from the—not all, but, you know, we picked names out of a phone book and all kinds of stuff like that. Anyway, it was a hard job, but we both filled our classes. I had mine in my studio and she had hers in her studio and then we exchanged the groups and finally we had them together. And that worked out very well. It was very exciting . . . she and I had a special relationship of talking to each other about what was going on and then trying to arrange this cross-disciplinary thing and running up against some snags about timing and personalities and the students and all kinds of stuff like that.

. . . at that point [we were] teaching colleagues. So that worked out well, and we did it again. I think we did it two or three times. By the time we offered it the third time, things had caught on. I mean, there were already other people doing something similar and some of the institutions had begun to have courses . . . finally it sort of petered out because we had tapped a very good vein of people and then, either there weren't many people left or they went off and found ways to continue their work or something.

. . . after that finished she was successful in starting her program because I know she was very serious about getting this started and was probably trying all along to do it. Now during that period, we were often invited by organizations to present at their conferences.

I remember one we did for a children's conference. They would invite us together, and we would work together . . . she would present the movement part, I would present the art part, we'd both talk and then we'd sum it up together. We were co-presenters. So that sort of grew out of our cooperation in doing this joint course.

Together Chapin and Ganet-Sigel began to educate the medical and psychiatric community about alternative or adjunct treatment modes. They began introducing art therapy and dance/movement therapy to the psychiatrists in the hospital setting. However, during this same time, as Chapin suggested, Don Sieden was the one person who was most responsible for bringing visual art therapy to the attention of the psychiatrists in Chicago. Chapin further explained the historical development of art and dance/movement therapies in the Chicagoland area.

. . . Jane was sending me interns. I actually had two dance therapists on my staff. . . . I was in such close contact with her. . . . Of course, she knew very, very well the two dance therapists that I had on my staff. . . . I think they were teaching for her. . . . [So Jane and I] would invite each other to teach at each other's classes. . . . If I wanted something for my class about dance movement, I would ask Jane and she would either send somebody or come herself. And she would invite me to do workshops for her students.

Lately, in the last few years, she was doing summer programs and invited me to do a day of art for the people enrolled in the summer programs in which the students got a taste of the various arts. And so she invited me to do the visual arts part which I did for a number of years until I left. Later I did a course — I was teaching then at the Art Institute — on empathy. And the course was for graduate students. I invited her to do one of the sessions, or a whole day, with my classes. And this happened a couple of times and of course, I told the program faculty at the Art Institute about her and her work, and she was sort of incorporated as a guest in her field in our program, as we were in hers. My students loved her, and she did a wonderful workshop with them. It was a great introduction for them. They were very, very receptive as you can imagine, just as her students were receptive to what I was offering.

Together Chapin and Ganet-Sigel played a major role in bringing art therapy and dance movement therapy respectively to the city of Chicago and the Midwest. They offered their insight, knowledge, and experience in the service of teaching others that there are different ways to understand and respond to clients' that the medical/therapeutic community otherwise had not considered.

I'm not saying we were the only ones, but we were the first really important teachers around there. We were pioneers. Except . . . for Don Sieden, who had his own work. As a result of our pioneering efforts, others' interest in both art therapy and dance/movement therapy just took off. We looked around the next year when we thought about doing the course again and looked at each other and said, "We don't think we need to do this, or we won't get enough students." Because they were all so busy with other things. There were in-services then in the various hospitals and courses here and there. I mean, it isn't that there weren't people who didn't know how to do this or teach it, but they were coming in from elsewhere. They were new people. The idea had caught on . . . with people like recreational therapists and occupational therapists and actually most of our classes at that point — I mean the courses that we did ourselves — were made up of occupational and recreational therapists who wanted to extend their know-how. And so they picked up a lot of techniques from us and began to use them. . . . Of course, they didn't have the full background in either of our disciplines, but they picked up a lot of techniques.

During this time Ganet-Sigel was already busy doing private practice work in her mother's basement, and planning the development of the graduate program in dance/movement therapy at Columbia College in Chicago.

Ganet-Sigel's Latter Career

Ganet-Sigel's latter career is comprised of her work as the program director, teacher, and then Chair of dance/movement therapy at Columbia College, her mentoring of young professionals, and her ongoing commitment to spreading the word about dance/movement therapy through national and international workshops.

Program director, teacher and mentor   From 1982–1998, Ganet-Sigel was the Director of the Graduate Program in Dance/Movement Therapy Program at Columbia College in Chicago. One of the goals of the program has been to develop practitioners who use movement to understand and facilitate client health. The program guided by the American Dance Therapy Association (ADTA) focuses primarily on helping students meet the following goals:

1. to acquire knowledge of theories, goals, techniques, and practice of dance/movement therapy.
2. to recognize the interrelatedness of environmental conditions, socio-cultural factors and emotional issues.
3. to acquire knowledge of the human body and how its processes affect development, expressive and communicative aspects of movement.
4. to apply techniques to the observation, analysis, assessment, and research of movement behaviors.
5. to promote an awareness and understanding of the dance/movement therapist's roles and functions according to the principles of psycho-social processes, cultural context and ethical behavior within facilities and environments that treat individuals, groups and families.

As an administrator, Ganet-Sigel's role included program development, community outreach, recruitment and retention of students, budgeting, scheduling, teaching, supervising, and mentoring students. During her tenure, the program at Columbia which has existed for 16 years has continued to expand while other programs were shrinking. At the time Jane assumed the chair's position, there were no jobs in dance/movement therapy. Since most students get jobs upon graduation, nowadays students can be assured that they will easily get a job when they're out of school. In fact many of their internship placements result in jobs upon graduation.

Describing how their relationship changed as she moved from her role as a student to colleague, one woman shared:

> [When I first met Jane she was my] teacher and mentor . . . and thesis supervisor. After graduation, she became my colleague. Sometimes we [have taught] together at Columbia; occasionally we've taught in the same classroom . . . We have written an article together [and] also made several conference presentations. One thing that's wonderful about Jane, as soon as her students graduate, they become her colleagues. She switches that whole thing, so you never feel like you'll always be her student, or you always know less. She treats you like a colleague, and you become her colleague the minute that you finish your work.

Another colleague shared:

> She's very open, and she's very supportive. And she has a lot of knowledge, and one thing about her that's really important is that, even though a lot of us have branched off . . . taken other trainings and we've added other things to our work . . . she stresses that we're dance therapists first, and we should remain pure in that and not become the other thing . . . when you're taking a new training, [even though] you want to embrace what they're doing and try it out on everything. . . . [Although] she's fine with all that adjunctive learning, she [always encouraged us] to be dance therapists first. And so [she] always kept me on track and . . . in the movement piece.

Another colleague recalled how supportive Ganet-Sigel was when she experienced difficult times working as a young therapist.

> . . . Jane has been there for me . . . in a lot of circumstances. There was a time I would consider myself a new therapist. I was in my first job out of graduate school. And I had a run-in with my supervisor. And basically, I got fired from the job. And it was one of those where I had just been written up as the best thing since sliced bread, so why was I being fired? Well, it's a long story, but there were moldy oranges in the cafeteria, and I said to the dietitian that there were some moldy oranges and I'm sure she wasn't aware of it, but . . .

> Anyway, I got written up on that, as did someone else . . . and they said that . . . if I could use poor judgment criticizing cafeteria food, that might spill over to my work with patients . . . at the time I was devastated. I couldn't understand. . . . I had just been written up for my work with a person that was a multiple personality . . . I ended up saving her life. . . .
>
> Later I discovered that this event was a political issue, and that they wanted to fire me and this other person because we were the highest paid people in our department. The whole hospital . . . had been changed . . . people that were in the department before me were trying to unionize. . . .

Fired over spoiled oranges, she went downtown to the National Labor Relations Bureau and said: "Look, you know, look at this. Oranges. I'm being fired over oranges. Look at this [write-up I just received from my supervisor telling what] a talented therapist [I am]." The National Labor Relations Board responded that they could not help her since she was not unionized. Ganet-Sigel's colleague continued:

> Anyway, so I called Jane . . . [and she was] was absolutely there for me . . . at the time, I remember thinking how much easier it would be to say, "I think I'll just go sell clothes or cosmetics or something where I don't have to use my mind, I can just go and do." You know? And, "Why do I want to do this?". . . I was learning, I was growing as a therapist, and all this other political crap that was happening around me I was really ready to just pack it in. And, you know, there was Jane, standing me up and talking to me and [saying], "What do you mean you're going to blah, blah, blah? You know the way Jane is.
>
> And she took over, and she absolutely backed me up. And [she said the] things I . . . needed to hear from her that . . . this is ridiculous. I needed to have someone get pissed off for me, with me and she was there. I mean, Jane can get pissed off like no one's business. But Jane was there [for me] . . . in terms of my growth as a therapist and my growth, as a person in relation to who I am as a professional, Jane has always been there. In many ways Jane has been my teacher, my friend, my mentor.

Another colleague shared how Ganet-Sigel became her colleague following a student's graduation.

> . . . we've worked all the way from teacher to colleague. And I did some therapeutic work with her, too, because I just found the work that she was doing to be so fascinating, and not only did it complement, I thought, what the music therapy work was doing but in some ways it made it even more in-depth.
>
> . . . When I went away . . . to New York for my internship after I finished up my training in Chicago. . . . I worked at a place called Creative Arts Rehabilitation Center, and there I really

found the work that I did with Jane to be a wonderful, wonderful preparation. We had music therapists, it was predominantly a music therapy place, but there were also dance movement therapists as well as art therapists. So it just was wonderful to have had her as a teacher and [to] have [had] that background.

. . . she's very convinced about what she does, and she does it with a great deal of passion. I think that's probably one of the things that really impressed me about her from the very beginning. She's convinced, but not convinced from simply a cognitive place. Her whole body knows what she teaches. I guess it should because that's what she's teaching . . . it's because of what Jane taught me that makes me really convinced that it's such a valid modality.

. . . As a teacher . . . she formed a whole generation of people who would carry on the dance movement therapy. And then I think I've seen her be a mentor, too, to people. I certainly look on her as a person who . . . has moved through the stages in her life to carry on with movement, for one thing. Because I think one of the things that we need to remember as creative arts therapists [is] that we need to be in relationship to our art. And so to watch her continue to do movement throughout stages of her life — not only in therapy but also for herself — I used to love to watch her move . . . is something that is really important to remember. I think the professionalism for me was to watch. That was a mentoring kind of thing.

. . . There was an integrity about the way she dealt with people, the way she applied her craft, if you will, the way she taught. That to me was an inspiration. You know, it's kind of like I could say that this woman held up the highest ideals and [that's an example of how] I would want to practice in my own work.

National and International workshops　Ganet-Sigel has presented numerous workshops and lecture/demonstrations throughout the country and internationally. A brief overview of some of her notable national workshop presentations follows.

In the same fashion that she nourished the development of dance/movement therapy in the Midwest, Ganet-Sigel also applied her skills as a gifted salesperson. For example, she has traveled to community colleges to teach students and faculty how the body and mind are related. Using a lecture/demonstration format, she has helped individuals understand how what they feel and think is reflected in their behavior and that their behavior often reflects unconscious feelings. Based on her work as a teacher and therapist, she offers audiences some examples from her work with others to show how the dance/movement therapy process can help integrate the mind and body.

In another workshop, she helped participants explore the range of dance/movement therapeutic techniques. During all day intensive workshops presented at the University of Wisconsin-Madison, participants had an experiential introduction to the movement process. They engaged in warm-up activities, and explored their space, textures, and their senses. In group activities they moved to words such as *swing, stretch, bounce, push* and *dodge*, or *bend, twist, shake, pull*, and *strike*. They also moved through the room in dyads and triads in response to words such as: *stars, sun, moon*; polarities (*feminine/masculine*). During a workshop presented at the Beck Center for Cultural Arts in Cleveland, participants engaged in mirroring, developmental progress of movements, primary movements, changing roles, and sculpting. These interactions were used to introduce participants to various movement techniques. Other related activities offered during this workshop included discussion, question and answer sessions, and an opportunity to present specific client issues and identify appropriate techniques.

Ganet-Sigel has also spoken to audiences about how specific techniques may be used to treat clients with a known psychiatric illness. During an interactive lecture/demonstration presented at the 1985 National Coalition for Arts in Therapy Association (NCATA) Joint Conference, she and another colleague invited participants to learn how to use dance/movement therapy techniques with private patients who suffer anorexia nervosa. In 1988, she gave a lecture/demonstration for the Midwest American Dance Therapy Association Conference to highlight the issues that impinge upon the role of dance/movement in the hospital and/or institutional setting versus private practice.

Around the world, Ganet-Sigel has conducted workshops in China, Mexico, and Argentina. In April 1993, at the invitation of a colleague Linda Cao, a former student, Ganet-Sigel and her husband Mel journeyed to China for a presentation she made at Beijing/Normal University. During this emotional and exciting journey, Ganet-Sigel recalled the challenge of working through language barriers. [After we arrived], "an incredible job of interpreting" by Linda Cao,[6] "with heads going back and forth like during a ping-pong game began." For the casual observer, these behaviors might have seemed rather amusing. Following her presentation and speech to a standing room only audience of graduate students in psychology and theater, she was bombarded with 3 hours of questions concerning Western psychology. During the next few days, Ganet-Sigel gave several workshops to over 30 people. Linda Cao, acting as interpreter, had an opportunity to observe the workshop participants' behavior. Linda reported how their behavior changed over two days of their work together. Behavioral changes ranged from "attitudes of defensive to curious, embarrassed to relaxed; excited: from giggling with each other to taking time to explore self; from questioning and confronting to sharing own feelings" (Ganet-Sigel, 1994, p. 71).

Throughout the workshops, cultural dispositions began to surface. For example, culturally ingrained habits and behaviors of ignoring indi-

---

[6] Linda Cao came from China four years ago. Linda achieved her B.A. and M.A. in Chinese Literature at Beijing Normal University and also taught Chinese Modern Drama there for two years. Linda was trained by famous Chinese Tai Chi and Chi Kong Masters in the Tai Chi program. Linda initially came to the United States to study comparative literature. However, when she learned about the dance/movement therapy program at Columbia College, she soon transferred. Linda completed her M.A. in Dance/Movement Therapy in May, 1993.

viduals and forgetting about oneself emerged. Although Chinese citizens are taught to hold their bodies in balance, they are not encouraged to move freely. These attitudes and actions were deemed appropriate for a nation that has built its legacy upon having people think and act together for the benefit of national growth and prosperity. Since China has now become more open, introducing dance/movement therapy is especially timely. The challenges imposed upon workshop participants when asked to move freely were eloquently illustrated by one individual who could not decide for himself how to move his own name.

As a nation, Chinese people have grown accustomed to behaving in accordance with the wishes and/or demands of authority figures. One Beijing Normal University student aptly summarized the experience of having had Ganet-Sigel's introduction to dance/movement therapy: "We have many foreign visiting professors lecture, but we never had such feelings like we experienced with Ganet-Sigel, she moved together with us, smiled together with us and shared together with us, we felt so close with her" (Ganet-Sigel, 1994, p. 71). Perhaps as a result of their experience with dance/movement therapy, China will begin to merge Eastern and Western psychology and explore the benefits of this therapeutic modality.

Ganet-Sigel has made presentations at the Instituto Integro in Guadalajara, Mexico, at the request of an expatriate colleague who left the United States and later established a dance/movement therapy program in Mexico. She conducted a week-long intensive study for students who were working towards a Master's degree in Gestalt therapy. Afterwards, she was invited to return to the Instituto Integro and offer another series of lectures/demonstrations. Subsequently she has served as a consultant to their program director in dance/movement therapy.

Upon learning about her pioneer work in dance/movement therapy and lectures/workshops with educational programs in China and Mexico, in 1994, the School of Yoga Foundation in Buenos Aires, Argentina invited Ganet-Sigel to present a lecture and workshop. Subsequently in 1996 she was invited once again to offer another series of lectures/demonstrations to students and faculty at the Brecha School of Movement and to work with the private practice patients of a colleague who was both a dance/movement therapist and a psychologist.

Traits of the Dance/Movement Therapist

By virtue of the work that they do, dance/movement therapists must have a tendency towards extroversion. The role of the dance/movement therapist requires that the individual be able to serve as a container for a client's innermost and sometimes intense feelings, and establish a secure environment that will foster a therapeutic alliance. What are the personality traits or dispositions that permit an individual to offer this kind of service? The ways that students, clients, colleagues, friends, and family members describe Ganet-Sigel provides insight into the answer to this question.

The personality dispositions of the therapist may be integrally connected to his/her ability to exemplify and facilitate Yalom's (1985) therapeutic factors. In his research concerning group psychotherapy therapeutic change, Yalom suggested that change occurs through a complex process and "intricate interplay of guided human experiences" (p. 3) that he identified as "therapeutic factors." The authors of this textbook suggest that the skills and behaviors demonstrated by therapist can be instrumental in facilitating therapeutic change. We use Yalom's therapeutic factors as a framework to portray characteristics that are essential to becoming an effective therapist. In this section we will explore how Ganet-Sigel's traits embody specific factors. An overview of the behaviors or events that exemplify the therapeutic factors include: developing altruism, facilitating corrective experiences within the family group, fostering group cohesion, encouraging interpersonal growth and learning, modeling imitative behavior, imparting information, promoting catharsis, instilling hope, embodying existential concerns, fostering universality, and developing social skills is presented.

Developing altruism Describing the relationship between her upbringing and her professional behavior, another colleague shared:

> We're talking here about [a woman that was not] from a privileged background, [a background] . . . that . . . also affirmed women's roles to . . . be submissive, [rather than] make a life of their own. Jane grew up during the Depression. Many of our contemporaries were not allowed to go to school beyond high school. They stayed at home and cared for the younger children. She did not come from those privileges [Ivy League school, professional expectations], but she certainly developed a vision for [what she wanted to do]. She did come from a tradition of service and caring and compassion and justice. [She was exposed to the idea of] following the rituals at home and yet [she was] exposed to the outer world, the excitement of learning and liberty of thought.
>
> [She was exposed to] a rich community life and a sense of belonging. Jewish ideals and values were things that people hung on to even though they tried to become assimilated in between two worlds. These roots, the things children learn . . . before they're three, the rituals of getting the house ready for Pesach, the changing of dishes, the special day of Shabbat, things can be special, things can be dedicated, no matter how much money you don't have. Judaism as a religion has never separated mind and body. And in the bones . . . in the generations of family life that she lived, [she] experienced the sense of values, the sense of caring and working in a community.

Facilitating corrective experiences within family groups Regarded as the matriarch of the family, she invites the whole family to come together for special events and strives to offer a sense of unity. One of her twenty-one grandchildren shared that:

> She has the whole family together. [At these times] I get to see all
> my cousins and aunts and uncles, and my parents, my grandpar-
> ents and everyone. She sort of holds the whole family together
> and the whole family is closer.

Offering her family members the gift of togetherness, one grandchild
pointed out how she has encouraged family members to stay in touch
with one another.

> . . . my sister, my cousin, and I, write on E-mail and we stay fair-
> ly abreast [and] in touch with each other. . . . I think a lot of [this
> is] because of the fact that my grandmother — also my grandfa-
> ther — have all kept the family doing things together and have
> kept us close as an extended family. Not all families are like that.
> And I think that that is a really neat gift.

A history of togetherness has catalyzed good feelings about family
celebrations. One grandson stated that: "I love getting together with
my family. It's one of the highlights of any holiday or sometimes even
just some day in the middle of summer or something."

Fostering group cohesion   Her love for family is evident in strong family bonds felt by her children and grandchildren. One of her children
theorized how her upbringing has probably influenced her beliefs about
the importance of family.

> Jane grew up with strong family, with strong belief in strong fam-
> ily and has gone on and maintained that philosophy in life and
> maintained pulling the family together. At certain times, it's a uni-
> fying feeling for a family which you don't always get. [All of us
> have gone off in] our different directions, as brothers and sisters
> and step-brothers and step-sisters, so oftentimes our lives get busy,
> [however] as we have our own kids and their activities as well as
> our own activities, [she still provides] those times that we get
> together. [I always experience these occasions as] nice times.
> Sometimes she's as much like an observer, like a little elf on a shelf
> somewhere in a corner just making sure that everybody's there
> and everybody seems to be enjoying the company of each other,
> interaction with each other. . . . So she provides the nest. And she
> has all the chickees come back, in a way.

Many people remarked about Jane's preference for good company rather than material things. Her husband, Mel, shared that
"Jane is ultimately charitable. She'd much rather have a good meal
with you and a nice quiet evening than a fur coat. She isn't into
material things. She is into the quality of the relationship and the
communication. . . ."

Also regarded as a consummate entertainer, one of her friends
remarked that she is a

wonderful homemaker. [She] doesn't think anything of having 40 people for dinner [and] wouldn't think of having anything less than 30 people. [She believes that] everyone who doesn't have a home should come [to her home]. Her door [is] always open. All her children would bring kids, it never rattles Jane. She's in complete control; nothing is too big for her.

Encouraging interpersonal growth and learning   Family, friends, and colleagues remarked about her boundless generosity. One of her grandsons recounted with humor one event that illustrates her desire to give to others.

> We had a barbecue one time, I think it was the Fourth of July, but it doesn't matter — and there were about twenty-five people coming. Jane and Mel were grilling chicken and hamburgers and hot dogs and I think, skirt steaks or something like that, there were four things. And she didn't know what anybody was going to eat, though, right? [However] she wanted to make sure she had enough food. Maybe everybody was going to come and they were going to want hot dogs or hamburgers or whatever. So what did she do? She went out and got two of everything for every person. That way she could be sure that nothing was going to run out. Mind you, some of these people were six year old kids!" [Some of the guests] were a few vegetarians, but she had two pieces of each thing for every individual.

Needless to say, Ganet-Sigel provided plenty of food that night. Her grandson continued: ". . . I didn't run out of food that day. You always go home with something. [You] never go home empty-handed from her house." Jane always sends her guests home with something to eat, plus the memories.

One of her children recalled fondly how Ganet-Sigel reached out to their teachers.

> Something that she did that was really nice growing up was [that] . . . every year she would have our teachers over for lunch one day during the spring at the end of the year. . . . [It] was really a nice thing for them, just really special. [Although] sometimes the dog would eat the lunch — we had one little dog in particular that would eat all the food.

One of her grandchildren shared that:

> She's possibly one of the most generous people that I think I've ever met. . . . She's always giving in some way or another—and always trying to help, if there's a problem or whatever. She's constantly sending gifts [for] every little holiday. For Valentine's Day, she sent me a gift, and [little things to acknowledge] Hanukkah. There's always something, always a gift. Whenever I call her, she yells at me for not reversing the charges on the phone on long distance rate.

> She has a little vacation, summer house thing in Union Pier, Michigan . . . and every summer she lets me go up there. My girl-friend and I go up there and stay for a week or so. And whenever [Jane and Mel] come and visit us, they take us out to dinner, and take us here or there. They won't let us pay for anything. They're so very generous, both Jane and Mel. . . . I don't know that that is totally unrelated to what she does, either. I mean, it seems like what she does is a sort of a . . . , I think any therapist is sort of generous. [It is a] generous sort of a profession . . . just helping people is a generous kind of thing.

However her generosity is just not about money, according to one of her grandsons.

> It's also about people. If she has Thanksgiving dinner and if there's somebody knows somebody in town — like Mel knew a man, a Polish man, who was here and didn't have any family, so he was invited to Thanksgiving. [Even though] he wasn't a member of the family and didn't really know anybody, he was invited. He came and shared the Thanksgiving dinner with us.

Her ability to give to others is an admixture of acknowledging others, making people feel welcome, listening, and being there for others. One of her grandsons remarked that:

> She definitely will listen . . . she's always willing to listen to you if you have a problem or you feel like, you just need somebody to talk to or whatever. A number of times, I've just sat down and talked with her about life issues, about tolerance . . . that's been my big life crisis in the last few years and being in [and out of] school and going back to school, and thinking of graduate school or whatever. But she's been there to talk to.

She is a person that many of her family members feel they can turn to in times of need. A grandchild stated:

> . . . Whenever I have a problem, if I feel like I need someone to talk to or whatever, she's somebody I feel like I can [go to]. Even though she says her opinion, others don't feel judged by it.

Expressing similar feelings a grandchild commented that: "absolutely not . . . it's an opinion, you know? She doesn't push it upon you. I suppose, [she just] offers it up, as it may be." Rather than second guess people, Ganet-Sigel makes her thoughts available so that people have choices. Concurring with this point of view, one of her grandsons commented that:

> She's always been very accepting of my girlfriends or whatever. I never like felt like I couldn't bring somebody or have somebody meet her or anything like that. Every card I get or whatever has

my girlfriend's name on it as well. That's really nice because it helps to feel like you're being accepted with somebody's family.

Another grandson shared one of his favorite stories about his grandmother's response to a homeless person who asked her for money. Ganet-Sigel told him:

> No, I will not give you money, but if you follow me into the store right here, I will buy you food. That is my grandmother's way of saying, "I can't tell you what to do, but it's my money to do with as I choose, and I'm going to buy you food because you tell me you're hungry." The man said *could I have food?* . . . And to make sure he didn't go buy alcohol with it, she bought him food. And I think that shows a lot about my grandmother. She's not going to tell you what to do, but if you ask for her help, she's going to try to show you the right path. I think she bought him enough food for a week. . . .
>
> She got a cart and they went down through the aisles and she bought him food. She bought him sandwiches, ready-made sandwiches from the deli. She bought him soda, water, chips. She bought him food. And I guess that's as I look at it, that's her way of saying, *There's the good and the bad.* If you ask for my help, I'm not going to help you do the bad. If you want my help, you've got to let me help you do the good . . . And when you ask for help, you're going to get help. But she's not going to help you in a way that's bad. She's going to help you in a way that [is for your own] good.

One of her close friends described her generosity in assuming the responsibility for hosting an impromptu party.

> I can tell you one incident that will stand out in my mind, and this will give you an idea what type of person Jane is. As I say, our children were very close in ages. In fact, two of each of our children were very, very, very close friends. My daughter was having her birthday, and years ago it was a big thing. I mean you'd have thirty, forty kids, you didn't take them out to Chucky Cheese, you didn't take them out to a gym or something. You had your party at home. And the day before the party, my two sons got the mumps. Well, I didn't know what to do. And Jane said, "You put a sign on the front door that the party's being held next door." We had the five-year-old's party next door with forty kids.

Also commenting about her generosity, one of her colleagues remarked that:

> . . . my experience with Jane is that she is extremely generous. She's very open. She's really an expanded human being. She's expanded into the universe, and she embraces everything that's there. And she interacts with it really well which hopefully somebody that's in that field can do, but that's not always true.

Even though she was in a position of authority, others did not feel constrained.

> But Jane has power — And she doesn't misuse it. Which I think is so — it's a beautiful thing. She's just generous of spirit, of love, of time, of listening, of speaking, and in being present with other people when they speak to her. Then she responds to them as a human being. Which, once again, she's really busy. She's got a lot to do, and I've never seen her like blow anybody off. She's right there with you, hears you, listens to you, and interacts with you.

Modeling imitative behavior   Ganet-Sigel's remarkable drive and perseverance was observed by several interviewees. One of her dear friends recalled that:

> When Jane started out, no one ever heard of dance therapy. I thought it was something that was created from nowhere. And she was my children's dance teacher. She had a dance studio here in Skokie. Very popular [with a] load of all the little kids, and she wasn't one of these kind of teachers that couldn't talk ballet to a three-year-old. She taught movement and coordination, and she had a very successful dance studio that both of my girls attended, along with half of Skokie. And then, of course, . . . she gave that up when she started going to school and started having a practice. . . .
>
> I said how in the heck is Jane going to do it with four kids? And she did. And she did a beautiful job managing both. . . . She was always, you know, anxious to get to the next rung in the ladder. She's fairly motivated and . . . if she had a goal, Jane did it, and finished it. She was never the kind that would take up knitting and leave half the sweater.
>
> Whatever Jane did, she finished, and she did well. She was an innovator. She was very aggressive. To do some of the things Jane did — I felt it was really . . . brave. To raise four children and go out and . . . develop a career is quite an accomplishment in those days. But Jane really put her career first. Yeah. I wouldn't say she put it ahead of her kids, but I would say it was very important to Jane. Very important. She had to give up a lot of time of her own to accomplish what she's had. She's got four wonderful children. And they're very secure individuals. So whatever she did, she did right. She did a good job. And she's always been a happy person. She was a wonderful daughter. She was a wonderful, wonderful daughter. She would never consider putting her parents in a nursing home. And if it meant the girl didn't show up, or she had to be over there to check on them or take them to the doctor and get everything, she did it. She was really a very giving daughter. And she had wonderful parents as well, so I don't think the apple falls too far from the tree.

Another friend remarked that she is a ". . . wonderful dancer, [an] Earth Mother persona." Acknowledging Ganet-Sigel's contributions to the field she commented that: "Certainly her work as a charter member and what she's done in the Midwest is phenomenal . . . how she has brought dance movement therapy to hospitals and nursing homes and special settings. She sort of single-handedly pioneered all the efforts." Stubbornness probably requires a similar type of energy that is found in an individual's drive and perseverance. According to one of Ganet-Sigel's grandsons, she exhibited this ability.

> My grandmother Jane is very stubborn. As she's gotten older, she's definitely gotten more open-minded. I'd say she's gotten much more liberal . . . she was never black and white but maybe then she believed so strongly in what was the better way, not necessarily the best way, but the better way to do things that if somebody didn't do it, she wouldn't get upset, but she'd be a little disappointed. [Essentially she would be saying,] I love you. I want you to do what's right. I don't want you to fall down again. And she really had to let people fall, but with your own family you don't want to see them fall. And she could be stubborn. [However,] Jane's a very secure woman. And she's controlling.

Regarding her capacity for growth, he also commented that: "She accepts her own imperfections, and she tries to become a better person every day by learning, by teaching instead of preaching."

Imparting information Regarded for her gift for teaching others about her profession as well as life, a friend of hers commented that Ganet-Sigel is:

> One of the warmest people anybody could ever meet. [She] is concerned with others feelings and helping them understand their feelings. [She] will offer help but pull back if not accepted. [She also] takes things very seriously, very deeply [and is] emotionally effected a great deal by the things she does. [Jane is] not the most easy-going person.
>
> She absorbed a second family, accepted [her husband] Mel's children as her own, tried to be very fair in her feelings towards them, to share herself with all of them evenly. She puts friends and family as high priorities for herself.

Respect for Ganet-Sigel's ability to communicate her thoughts is shared by others. One of her children commented that:

> She's very strong-willed and opinionated. People sometimes get offended by her because she is so opinionated, but I think that it is just her opinion. Some people get offended because they take things personally.

Others discussed her capacity for empathy. One friend shared that she is:

> an unbelievable giving individual [and] very capable. She has an unbelievable ability to put herself in your place. She can feel what you're going through. Her capacity to empathize [is remarkable]. [She is] definitely a modern woman, very motivated. [She is] an innovator; brave.

Ganet-Sigel has a strong commitment to family. She is well known for her attempts to bring the family together. She is a communicator who strives to see the good side of things. She is very caring and loving about her family and others. One of her children characterized her as a person that likes to give.

> She gives freely of her time. She likes to get things and give things to people. Sometimes we laugh, because . . . she buys things that nobody needs. Her children and grandchildren kind of laugh during holiday time because she buys some really weird gifts for some of us. But we all know that she buys them for us because she wants you to share the pieces of her experience in foreign countries. I mean, she'll buy us all these hats that nobody in their right mind would wear from Bali or we have whole garage sales of things that she's given all of us.
>
> And we laugh when we open Hanukkah presents because if one person gets a weird hat, we know everybody else is going to get one. They buy by the dozen. [Jane and Mel] buy eleven of something or twelve or eighteen of something wherever they go. And there's a piece of that generosity that's really wonderful . . . you have to remember to keep this outlook on it that she's really caring and loving. . . . I know she got it because she cares about us, but we really — it's not something we're going to use.

Her attentiveness to her children and grandchildren was observed by family members and colleagues. Another one of her children commented:

> She is a very emotionally attentive individual. That certainly blossomed amongst not only her children but her grandchildren which continued to multiply. And each have been given a special and individual relationship with her, which, for the grandkids is really something special that you don't often or always see with grandparents. [She gives each one] very specific loving.

She is regarded by her children for the way in which she acknowledges people and makes everybody feel welcome as an individual. However one of her children suggested that she was somewhat overbearing. "Her attentiveness can at times certainly be too attentive. We have to tell her to close the valve a little. She probably raised all of us to be moderately opinionated, but it's always with great intentions."

Her grandchildren regard her attentiveness with fondness. If they are in a play or in a concert, Ganet-Sigel likes to come and see them perform. She also takes them out to celebrate special times. One of her granddaughters remarked:

> She'll always ask when's your concert or when's this event, let me know or whatever and then . . . she won't get really mad [if we forget to tell her and she will say something like], "You didn't tell me." I know she likes to see us do our activities and everything.

Her granddaughter also shared:

> Well, ever since I can remember when [I was] little, for each one of my birthdays she would have us come over for our birthday and sleep over at her house for one night around our birthday. And then the next morning or that evening she used to take us shopping. I liked to go to Toys R Us when I was little. And she'd let us spend fifty dollars and, you know, get the toys we wanted or whatever. . . . She's pretty caring [and] interested in my life. . . .

One of her colleagues commented that the close relationships that develop between her and her co-workers are

> . . . due to her being supportive and sensitive to others . . . [she] nurtures personal growth, honesty [and] appreciation for the individual. As a colleague [she] provides a listening ear as a resource really for bouncing things off. [Jane] . . . empathizes, [offers] understanding versus judging, and caring respect for people.

Another one of her colleagues described her commitment to family.

> She's a very family-oriented person and draws a lot of strength by being that way. She is the family matriarch. Her close family ties give her a lot of nurturance and strength that she needs in order to do so much giving with clients and students.

Promoting catharsis   Ganet-Sigel has a facility to speak her mind and say how she believes it is. She is regarded as a loving woman who will freely speak her mind but will respect others' viewpoints. A friend of hers commented that Ganet-Sigel is:

> [She is] adored and respected by her family. [Jane] will voice her viewpoint but acknowledge if a friend's doesn't agree with her and that doesn't hinder the friendship in any way.

One of her children remarked:

> Well, she's I would say, very opinionated. Very . . . confident and has her own mind. Yet I think she's very compassionate to other people's viewpoints . . . you feel like you can be heard and

acknowledged, but she'll also share with you what she's feeling and thinking, too.

Instilling hope   As a individual, she is regarded as a strong and centered person. One colleague described her as:

> . . . the rock of Gibraltar; that's my image of her. She's a very centering kind of person, solid, and grounded. It's a rare thing to have someone in your life that you know when you that they'll be there for you and they'll be supportive. [She] always takes time. If you have a problem, she always takes time to listen to you and she's very helpful. You can draw on her not just as a teacher, but as a friend and support person.

One of her friend shared that: "Jane has an embracing aura, a physical warmth that pervades the interchange. Her presence bespeaks that primitive human bonding . . . the very reason why dance therapy works with people." One of her grandsons commented:

> She's just remarkable [in how] she deals with [things] professionally and personally. I mean, she has her private practice. She's the director at Columbia College. She'll help anybody."

One of her students concurred with that impression and stated that: "[She is a] role model, friend. I can reach Jane for any kind of help." Another student commented:

> [she is a]very rich and complex person [who] didn't put up with a lot of bullshit. [She had] strength of character [and] wasn't afraid to say anything. I always knew where I was with her. [I] liked Jane [and] loved her as a teacher and as a friend. [She is a] real person you could bounce off against. [She] wasn't fake. I think it's very refreshing to find someone who's so real.

One other student remarked that although some students would at times complain about her, at other times the same students could be heard saying:

> When I get older, I'd like to be like Jane, so active, energetic, and so sharp. They all love her, adore, and admire her. She's a role model for us.

Another student shared that "[I] just really loved Jane. [Jane] supported students who wanted to go into other avenues that they had a passion for . . ."

Embodying existential concerns   Describing the energy that is felt from her, one colleague shared:

> [Jane epitomizes] the example of a woman with a fully developed professional life, a fully developed personal and family life, with all of its struggles, struggling through it all yet maintaining this sort of this love for — I admit it's a little bit cliché-ish, but she had a real energy and love for life . . . here's a woman in her seventies and just still going strong with all of it. Feeling the fatigue of it but sort of treasuring. I kind of feel her treasuring it all. . . . There's an energy and a will that just exudes from her whole being. . . . The eyes twinkle. And I feel it more and more as she ages. And she's aging well. And I sometimes look at her and like laugh . . . she's like this — sort of this living, moving Buddha who sort of exudes this — oh, wisdom and energy and love and good will. And that's not to say she doesn't have other sides to her, too, and that's why I really want to emphasize the humanness—in the visceral sense.

Another friend concurred:

> The first time I met her, I saw the twinkle in her eye. And how many years ago was that already? And I recall when my husband first met her, just to say hello to her, when we were engaged. The first thing he said to me is, Her eyes twinkle. You could see it in her eyes, and it's like this little elf. Of course, she's not an elf in her presence, but there's something in her viscera that communicates passion through her whole being and it exudes. You feel it.

Another colleague described her as a mensch.

> I guess there's a word — a mensch? A jewel of a person . . . that includes the whole of her humanness. She's a very human person. . . . I really want to emphasize that, because she has been such a figurehead for people in the field of dance therapy, both good and bad, in the midwest. And that through it all there has been on her part, just a warmth and a love of people, of relationships. I'm just very aware of her nurturing of relationships, as I work in the office. Her nurturing of the staff, her feeding of everybody, both literally and figuratively.

Fostering universality Many colleagues shared their characterizations of Ganet-Sigel.

> I think Jane has gone through a tremendous amount in terms of pioneering. . . . She's put on her little bonnet in front of her covered wagon. . . . I think that she has gone through a tremendous amount in terms of pioneering in this field, not just in Chicago but I think in the field in general . . . I think that Jane is a very talented therapist . . . in terms of working with what she lovingly calls "normal neurotics" in private practice, I think she can't be surpassed. I think she is intuitive [and] has the ability to very gently and not so gently prod, push, get angry, hug, hold, love

and elicit trust that I think we all feel for her. I think she's an incredible human being.

Jane Ganet-Sigel has touched a multitude of lives ". . . both personally as well as professionally, she has touched a lot of people's lives in a very, very profound way." Another colleague stated that: "She's an amazing person. You don't need much contact with her to be impressed with what she does. She has a charisma that is quite unique." Another colleague commented:

> She's one of those people who is able to be so clear and direct and set goals and steps to achieve them. She gets them going, and also she is a very, very sensitive therapist. She really is a remarkable woman. She's not self-aggrandizing either. She's a person who I think she knows herself, she has a mission, but she's not blatant about it. I think she enjoys what she does. And she certainly has made an enormous difference in this area, the Chicago area, for the creative arts therapy. She has students and interns all over.

Suggesting the way that Ganet-Sigel's work in the field of dance/ movement therapy should be characterized, one colleague stated:

> [She is an] extraordinary human being. You could use the word "totemic." [Jane] challenges mediocrity. [She is] is someone who has vision, who is a mover and a shaker. She's got conviction. She needs to be placed up there with the Chaces, Whiteheads, and other people like Chaiklin and others who have put themselves up there. It's time for her to get her accolades.

Another colleague reported :

> I think Jane is a visionary. And she had a beautiful vision about what it means to be in touch with your body and what that means in terms of what it could do for your life and what you can process with your body . . . she manifested that vision which is basically what the department chairs at Columbia are [like]. They're huge visionaries who have created something — it's not like they took something somebody else did and changed it, but they created something out of their own vision. Jane is one of those people who have done that. I think that this is something with visionaries that sometimes they're also very controlling. [However] Jane is unusual in that she is a visionary. . . . She is able to let other people participate in the vision which I think is a very unusual trait . . . She's greatly loved by the people around her. She's warm and generous and kind and open and loving and not controlling which I think is really beautiful.

Recognizing Ganet-Sigel's unique talents, this colleague commented:

I think Jane is an artist as well as being a really visionary person who then creates something that is practical. So she's really a good mix of practicality and visionary, which is also unusual. But that's why she's been able to build a program that has as much power as it has. . . . Jane knows that the gifts that she's been given . . . belong to everybody, and she's the vehicle for that manifestation. . . . She's worked hard to manifest and has manifested very well . . . she's not some powerful God-owner of something or other. I think Jane is very humble.

Describing Ganet-Sigel's humanity, a colleague shared:

We've gone on long walks together. And we've sat on the stools of restaurants at very cheap little hash houses that [were] very good and eaten eggs and canned peas together. But I would say that the thing that I've experienced most with her . . . is the respect with which she treats other people like when we're having a meeting.

. . . I just really like the way she is in a meeting. She just really lets people be who they are and listens to them. And she doesn't cut anybody off. [I have observed] Jane's ability to lay back and just enjoy life. She can let go and just sit back and watch and just enjoy what's around her.

Developing social skills   One of her colleagues, a former student shared:

. . . from this vantage point, I can appreciate the great courage it took for her as . . . a lone woman, in a sense, to premier that field in the Midwest . . . when I said from this vantage point . . . at the other end, we always thought of her as this staunch person. At this end, I can see how hard that was, and that in many ways she didn't put herself forward, . . . in the academic realm or ask for things as much as she might have. So there's this dual view that I'm trying to communicate to you. At one end, Jane is sort of this strong person who is outspoken, and yet from this end, . . . I see her as really very sensitive.

Ganet-Sigel's ability to serve as a mentor was also recalled. One colleague shared:

I haven't had many female examples or mentors that I can really respect. And she somehow embodies it all. There's a femininity to her in the ultimate sense . . . which I think . . . that students come to respect . . . we're largely a female community, but one of the things that she really stresses is that you have to go on in the midst of it all, that life goes on in the midst of it all. And that you have to go along with it, you have to embrace life.

Making a commitment to create an awareness and understanding of a field takes tremendous inner strength and resources. Ganet-Sigel acknowledges how the love and support of family and friends helped her persevere.

> . . . personally [I] was guided by and could not get to this stage without the poetry and romance for life that my father gave me [and] the control, energy and sweetness from my mother. The part my ex-husband played in helping me produce four beautiful children. My children, whose understanding of my involvement with people, humor and sensitivity has always been there.

The responses of many individuals have helped keep her grounded throughout the years.

> The exhilaration and love of my grandchildren, my extended family, brother, sister-in-law, and dear friends, their love and pride in me, my students' and clients' trust and belief in me, and above all, my present husband's willingness to flow through struggles with me, [his] understanding of dance/movement therapy, support, love, and bringing even more lovely children and grandchildren into my life [had refueled my energies].

Conclusion

As we have seen, Ganet-Sigel embodies many aspects of Yalom's therapeutic factors:

developing altruism   to learn that one can be regarded as useful to others.

facilitating corrective experiences within the family group   to challenge maladaptive behavior patterns and to replace them with more healthy behaviors.

fostering group cohesion   to bring about a sense of affiliation and belongingness.

encouraging interpersonal growth and learning   to gain insight about self and others.

modeling imitative behavior   to learn new behaviors by observing others.

imparting information   to help others develop insight into dance/movement therapy and human behavior.

promoting catharsis   to learn how to express feelings freely while respecting others.

instilling hope   to remain optimistic, maintain strong convictions, and a sense of faith.

embodying existential concerns   to transform destabilizing events and feelings into growth inducing experiences.

fostering universality   to recognize that there exists a commonality among individuals' felt experiences.

developing social skills   to learn how to interact with others in adaptive and healthy ways.

Hopefully this framework will inspire further exploration between Yalom's therapeutic factors and the essential skills and behaviors of an effective therapist.

Many books have been written about dance/movement therapy: Chaiklin (1984); Espenak (1981); Lefco (1974); Lewis (1984); Lewis (1986); Mason (1974); Payne (1992); Sandel, Chaiklin & Lohn (1993); Schoop (1974); Siegel (1988); and Young (1986). These texts in addition to Levy's textbook (1988) which provides an excellent historical account of the field, offer limited research and discussion about the exhaustive efforts of Ganet-Sigel among others in the Midwest to educate and promote dance/movement therapy. As one family member stated:

> She's really worked very hard and very diligently in the field and to try to make it something respectable here in the Midwest, Chicago area in particular. It would be nice to see her get more recognition for that . . . beyond the local area, where she has the name and people know who she is.

One of her former students, now a practicing dance/movement therapist, remarked:

> What's going to make Jane be alive in people's memories and understand what a hell of a job she has done, what she has come through, is to know all of the things, all of the obstacles that were set in front of her by the people that were supposed to be supporting her efforts.

Ganet-Sigel has had a seminal role in the emergence of dance/movement therapy in the Midwest and Chicago. Without her pioneering efforts, it is difficult to assess whether or not the field would have become recognized as a viable alternative to help patients heal themselves. The dearth in historical accounts of the field are underscored by several events. First, the legacy of her contributions to the field up to this point have been primarily undocumented. Second, there has been no single work written about the therapist's role in working with outpatients. Another interesting facet of this account relates to the innovative role and unique journey that this woman experienced.

Jane Ganet-Sigel is regarded by people who know her as a leader among women as both a professional and as an individual. Raised in an era when women had been socialized to take care of children, remain in the home, care for their spouse and behave submissively, Ganet-Sigel went out, started a new career, opened a private practice at the age of nearly fifty, and founded a graduate program in dance/movement therapy at the age of 56. These remarkable undertakings for a single woman and mother of 4 children took courage and perseverance. The mere fact she had the vision to promote her profession to people in the medically affiliated community was astounding and remarkable.

CHAPTER 3

Teaching the Foundations of Dance/Movement Therapy

Guiding Questions

1. *Why is it important for teachers of dance/movement therapy to plan for instruction?*

2. *How can teachers of dance/movement therapy design instruction that is responsive to students' varied learning styles?*

3. *How can a knowledge of teaching models be used?*

4. *According to the authors, what are the characteristics of effective teachers of dance/movement therapy?*

5. *In what ways can an understanding of the characteristics of adult learners be helpful to teachers of dance/movement therapy?*

6. *How do field-dependent and field-independent students differ in their approach to learning?*

7. *How has Ganet-Sigel helped students translate classroom learning experiences to practice?*

8. *What models of teaching does Ganet-Sigel use?*

Teachers for the 21st century need to have an array of tools that will permit them to make conscious decisions about their teaching (Behar-Horenstein, 1994). He or she must understand the structures of subject matter, the principles of conceptual organization, and the principles of inquiry . . . (Shulman, cited in Ornstein and Behar-Horenstein, 1999, p. 109).

We find few analyses of teachers that give careful attention not only to the management of students in classrooms, but also to the management of ideas in classroom discourses (Shulman, cited in Ornstein and Behar-Horenstein, 1999, p. 103). Each teacher's story seeks to impart something of a practical nature regarding how that particular teacher copes with instructional and curricular matters in the context of his or her environment (Behar-Horenstein, cited in Ornstein and Behar-Horenstein, 1999, p. 97). It is the wisdom of practice itself that guides . . . the practices of able teachers (Shulman, cited in Ornstein and Behar-Horenstein, 1999, p. 111).

The dance/movement therapist-teacher must carefully consider how to integrate the content, processes of learning, and social climate when developing curriculum for classroom teaching. As a teacher, the dance/movement therapist must determine how content will be taught and how it will be conveyed. The components of the learning and instructional process that need to be considered include: (1) determining how students learn best, (2) matching students' learning and thinking styles with instruction, and (3) identifying appropriate models of teaching to guide planning and instruction. The social climate of the classroom/clinical environment will be influenced by the type of structure that the teacher selects, the students' and teacher's demeanor, and the quality of interactions between students and teacher.

To address these topics, the authors have divided this chapter into four sections. First, they offer a framework for developing curriculum and course syllabi for dance/movement therapy students. In this section they provide an overview of related topics, (1) developing a plan for teaching, (2) using models of teaching, (3) teaching to students' learning styles, (4) developing goals for all students, and (5) demonstrating interpersonal skills. Second, after a brief description of the characteristics of the adult learner, they provide an overview of the individuals who choose to study dance/movement therapy. In the third section, in the context of Joyce and Weil (1996), they analyze and identify Ganet-Sigel's use of teaching models. In this section the following question is considered. How does Ganet-Sigel help students translate theoretical concepts into therapeutic strategies? The authors discuss how classroom experiences influence the actual training of a therapist. Additionally they describe how Ganet-Sigel helps students translate theoretical concepts and textbook learning into therapeutic strategies for use in outpatient and hospital settings with a variety of clients. In the final section, they describe how she successfully trained a seventy-year-old dancer to become a dance/movement therapist.

Developing Curriculum and Course Syllabi

Crucial to course development is identification of central or important questions that help delimit what is most fundamental to the dance/movement therapy curriculum. Formulation of these questions also ensures maintenance of the scope and coherence of a curriculum. Once these questions have been identified, the instructor will be able to determine the specific course objectives. Identifying both the focus and objectives of a course syllabus is an important activity that requires conscious decision-making about curriculum development. These processes empower the dance/movement therapist-teacher to make informed and rational choices about the what and how he/she plans to teach and increases the likelihood that instruction will be focused and well thought-out.

The goal of classroom/clinical teaching is to make students explicitly aware of what is expected of them as a result of the instructional

Table 3.1   A FRAMEWORK TO GUIDE CURRICULUM PLANNING AND COURSE DEVELOPMENT IN DANCE/MOVEMENT THERAPY

1. What competencies should dance/movement therapy students attain?
2. What type of learning experiences will help dance/movement therapy students attain competencies?
3. What curriculum modifications will be necessary to accommodate the students' individual needs?
4. What evidence is there to confirm that dance/movement therapy students have attained the desired competencies?

process, help them see the relevance and connectivity of learning experiences to their work as a practitioner, and build their expertise and confidence as a skilled dance/movement therapist. However in acknowledgment of the growing diversity and pluralism of college-age students, it is important to consider what their particular learning needs and styles may require from the teacher. The framework shown below (see Table 3.1) can be used to guide curriculum planning and the development of syllabi in dance/movement therapy courses.

Developing a Plan for Teaching

Developing a plan for teaching is integral to successful student outcomes. Planning, considered to play a central role in the professional activity of teachers, guides what is taught in classrooms. Teachers must carefully balance several variables when engaged in planning including subject matter and competencies, student needs, the learning environment, and personal preferences. For example, teachers must make decisions about the pace, scope and sequence of learning activities. They must decide how much time to spend on a topic, as well as what additions or deletions should be made to the course curriculum.

To ensure that students understand what is expected, teachers must convey explicitly to students what they should be able to demonstrate at the end of a unit or course. Thus it is incumbent upon teachers that they are capable of developing distinct ideas and/or visual representations of the changes in students' behavior that they seek to elicit as a result of their instruction. Learning activities should be selected and sequenced so that they coincide with the intended learning objectives. Also, students need ample time to practice and experience behaviors or skills to increase the likelihood that they will be successful in acquiring competencies. For example, students should have adequate amounts of guided practice so that the professor can monitor their progress as well as individual practice so that they can work independently with newly acquired or emerging skills.

Helping students to become their own gatekeepers in attaining new knowledge is one of the goals in training the aspiring dance/movement therapist. Essential to this goal is developing metacognitive strategies, which can be defined as "learning how to learn." This is a crucial activity in becoming a self-regulated and independent learner whereby students can pursue topics of self-interest on their own and make sense of the material they study. Moreover, the quantity of skills and information that students might acquire is often not nearly as important as experiencing depth and breadth in a particular content and learning process skills. Placing an emphasis on depth rather than the amount of material may encourage students to make inquiry into related topics of interest and transfer skills to other subject matter.

Using Models of Teaching

Each time instructors enter the classroom, their teaching is generally consciously or unconsciously guided by some model of teaching. Some instructors use models of teaching explicitly; others may not use them consciously. Yet some teachers enter the classroom without a well-thought out plan or clear ideas of what they hope to accomplish during instruction. What are models of teaching? Models of teaching are conceptual frameworks used by teachers that help students learn how to learn. Joyce and Calhoun (1996) have suggested that models of teaching are really models of learning. They have classified these models into four families: information-processing, social, personal, and behavioral systems approaches.

The information processing models focus on enhancing students' ability to make sense of their work by acquiring and organizing information, identifying and solving problems, and learning concepts. These models are designed to promote students' awareness of strategies that can help them make inquiry into, and reflect upon, the world. This family of models focuses on helping students learn how to construct knowledge (see Table 3.2).

Instructors select information processing models when they are trying to impart a new concept or an idea to students and provide situations in which they may identify the concept or idea in action. Within this framework, dance/movement therapy students could learn about the theories and techniques of dance/movement therapy through readings, lectures, and student participation. They may focus on identifying elements that are common to all dance/movement therapy techniques and the different and specialized techniques used to meet the needs of various pathologies and special population groups.

The social family of models uses the synergy of group interactions to build learning communities. These models encourage students to construct knowledge through group inquiry and use problem-solving strategies as they learn to participate in democratic processes. Students learn to use their awareness of personal and social values to address issues related to patient care (see Table 3.3).

The social models are used to encourage students to use scientific, social, and other relevant knowledge to make decisions about clinical

Table 3.2 Information-Processing Models*

MODEL	PURPOSE
Inductive Thinking	To classify information and concepts, build conceptual understanding of disciplines, and learn to build and test hypotheses based on classifications.
Concept Attainment	To learn specific concepts and strategies to attain them, gain control over subject matter, build hypotheses and study thinking.
Scientific Inquiry	To acquire scientific process, knowledge bases, and major concepts of specific disciplines. Conceptual thinking, hypothetical reasoning and ability to think critically are developed.
Inquiry Training	To learn how to reason causally, collect data, build concepts, and develop and test hypotheses.
Cognitive Growth	To increase intellectual growth.
Advanced Organizer	To increase ability to synthesize and organize information from multiple sources.
Mnemonics	To develop strategies for mastering new concepts, facts, and ideas.
Synectics	To use analogies to develop creative capacity.

* = Adapted from Joyce and Calhoun, 1996. CREATING LEARNING EXPERIENCES: THE ROLE OF INSTRUCTIONAL THEORY AND RESEARCH. Alexandria, VA: Association for Supervision and Curriculum Development. pp. 10–11

Table 3.3 Social Models*

MODEL	PURPOSE
Group Investigation	To reflect upon one's self and one's own values, develop a commitment to improving society, and participate productively in a democracy.
Social Inquiry	To work together to solve social problems, and develop strategies for problem-solving.
Jurisprudential Inquiry	To analyze issues of public interest using a legal framework.
Laboratory Method	To develop strong and sensitive social skills while learning how to understand group dynamics.
Role Playing	To learn strategies for resolving conflict and social problems.
Positive Interdependence	To learn how to work together interdependently and appreciate the nature of self-others relationships.
Structured Social Inquiry	To learn to work together cooperatively in the pursuit of academic inquiry.

* = Adapted from Joyce and Calhoun, 1996. CREATING LEARNING EXPERIENCES: THE ROLE OF INSTRUCTIONAL THEORY AND RESEARCH. Alexandria, VA: Association for Supervision and Curriculum Development. pp. 13–14

Table 3.4 Personal Models*

MODEL	PURPOSE
Nondirective Teaching	To build capacity for self-development and create personal awareness.
Awareness Training	To enhance personal growth through self-understanding, increasing empathy, and sensitivity towards others.
Classroom Meeting	To increase responsibility to self and others. To increase self-understanding.
Self-Actualization	To increase capacity for personal development and self-understanding.
Conceptual Systems	To increase one's own flexibility in interacting with others and propel individuals to higher levels of conceptual development as they learn to process information.

* = Adapted from Joyce and Calhoun, 1996. CREATING LEARNING EXPERIENCES: THE ROLE OF INSTRUCTIONAL THEORY AND RESEARCH. Alexandria, VA: Association for Supervision and Curriculum Development. p. 15

situations or dilemmas with patients which may have personal, social, or political implications.

According to Joyce and Calhoun (1996), the personal family of models emphasize helping students become self-actualizing, self-aware, and able to direct their own destinies. An instructor will use this family of models when utilizing a non-directive teaching style. This approach helps students explore their own existential goals or reflect upon the things that he or she would like to do in their career. Students taught using the personal family of models demonstrated an increased capability to learn (see Table 3.4).

The behavioral family of models relies extensively on developing student mastery in the acquisition of new knowledge. Students are also encouraged to adapt their behavior and to make changes that will bring about desired outcomes. The behavioral family of models is used to guide student learning in which success or outcomes are measured by their ability to demonstrate new behaviors (see Table 3.5).

How does the use of a teaching model benefit instructors and students? How does the explicit use of a teaching model guide practice and student outcomes? How is teaching affected when an instructor does not use a coherent model to guide instruction? Joyce and Weil (1996) suggest that the explicit use of teaching models can accelerate students' rate of learning and lead to increased measures of academic achievement for all students. Teaching models are also an important component in increasing students' capacity and facility in learning (Joyce and Calhoun, 1996). As students' repertoire of learning strategies increases, they change and can accomplish more types of learning effectively. Increasing students' aptitude ... "is a fundamental purpose of teaching models" (Joyce and Calhoun, 1996, p. 19). Choosing among an array of teaching models ensures that the best

Table 3.5 Behavioral Systems Models*

MODEL	PURPOSE
Social Learning	To develop an understanding of one's own behavior and its consequences. To develop more adaptive behaviors in order to attain goals.
Mastery Learning	To master content in all subject areas.
Programmed Learning	To master academic content. To help students monitor their own growth and modify learning strategies.
Simulation	To apply problem-solving concepts and problem-solving skills in situations that approximate realistic conditions.
Direct Teaching	To master academic content, enhance motivation and learn how to pace one's self.
Anxiety Reduction	To learn how to control aversive emotions and avert dysfunctional responses.

* = Adapted from Joyce and Calhoun, 1996. CREATING LEARNING EXPERIENCES: THE ROLE OF INSTRUCTIONAL THEORY AND RESEARCH. Alexandria, VA: Association for Supervision and Curriculum Development. p. 17

possible learning experiences can be selected for each purpose and each group of students.

A teacher's selection of a model is influenced by his/her perception of the nature of content and how it is best taught, and in turn influences the selection of the learning strategies that will facilitate successful outcomes and the quality of social interactions that are appropriate for classroom learning. Whether the content will be conceptual or contextualized, whether the process of teaching will be passive or constructive, and whether the social climate will be interactive or restrictive depends upon the model of teaching selected (Joyce and Calhoun, 1996). Designing appropriate learning experiences is a central concern of the teacher. Research has shown that methods of teaching influence what is learned and how well it is learned (Joyce and Calhoun, 1996). Certain methods increase desired outcomes; other methods diminish intended outcomes. By using models of teaching, we are really teaching students how to learn. Learning how to learn is crucial to perpetuating self-regulated and independent learners. Joyce and Calhoun (1996) claim that: "... the most important long-term outcome of instruction may be students' increased capacity to learn more easily and effectively in the future, both because of the knowledge and skills they have acquired and because they have mastered the learning process" (p. 6).

Models of teaching comprise major philosophical and psychological orientations towards teaching and learning. The use of teaching models also reflects an educator's philosophy, that is, how he or she believes students learn best and what knowledge is worth most. Moreover, the selection of the teaching model reflects an educator's perceptions of what content should be selected and how learning activities should be sequenced to help students meet desired instructional goals. Finally, the selection of a teaching model also reflects the ways in which educators believe that outcomes or student products ought to be evaluated. When choosing a model, the teacher must take into account the type of learning that will take place as well as the students' learning style. Teaching adults has a different set of implications and requirements than teaching children.

We know that if a teacher enters a classroom and repeatedly uses only one model of teaching, this is analogous to the artist using the same palette of colors. This behavior is likely to limit the scope of their creativity and the development of students' potential.

When selecting a model of teaching several factors must be considered. First, teachers must have a clear idea about what kind of knowledge they are trying to impart. What type of orientation will the lesson emphasize? For example, will the lesson focus on understanding (declarative knowledge), such as knowing, or acquiring new ideas, facts, principles, theories and generalizations? Will the lesson focus on skill-building and learning how to demonstrate mental abilities (procedural knowledge) such as problem solving, interpretation, analysis, application, or modeling a physical ability? There are several orientations associated with the design of learning experiences, including inquiry, appreciation, problem-solving, decision, skills, and personal growth.

The inquiry orientation aims at understanding. In learning activities that emphasize this orientation, the teacher and student may explore topics to search for underlying reasons, meanings, or implications of an event. For example, dance/movement therapy students may investigate the purpose or utility of various theoretical approaches and assessment techniques and discuss how they influence the development of patient treatment plans. Students may also explore questions such as:

1. What is the structure and function of Laban notation?
2. How can Laban notation be used to assess a patient's movement repertoire?

Appreciation-oriented learning experiences help students learn to identify personal preferences and criteria for making choices. When engaged in learning activities that are related to this orientation, students might weigh their preference for working in private practice versus hospitals or special education facilities based upon the quality of these respective environments.

The problem-solving orientation focuses on developing students' ability to solve problems. This might be accomplished by role play activities that students experience during in-class group simulations. Role playing involves creating authentic analogies to real-life therapeutic situations. During this experience, students are encouraged to observe, understand, and resolve experience-based problems. Students' feelings may be revealed during the role play. Revelation of personal feelings can be used to explore how they influenced the student's resolution of a therapeutic problem or selection of an intervention.

Students can also analyze this material during periods of private reflection. Role playing encourages students and/or the dance/movement therapist-teacher to examine how one's own feelings, attitudes, values, and beliefs impact enactment.

Decision-oriented learning experiences provide students with information or frameworks to use when weighing the advantages and disadvantages associated with particular decisions. Deciding where to set up a practice and identifying the populations of clients to work with are some of the determinations that dance/movement students will need to make.

Learning experiences that promote a skills orientation emphasize the acquisition of technical abilities or improving performance in carrying out physical tasks. Learning how to mirror a client's movement is an example of a behavior associated with a skills orientation.

Learning experiences that encourage personal growth are designed to help students define personal goals, focus on self-actualization, and develop a way to work toward that goal. During the process of becoming a dance/movement therapist, students learn how to separate their own issues from the client's, so that they can remain fully attuned to the client's needs. They may also need to cope with receiving critical feedback regarding their work. The successful resolution of these challenges is likely to catalyze personal growth.

The teacher must also consider the kind of environment he or she wishes to establish: a highly structured situation in which the teacher dominates instruction, a moderately dominated structure in which teacher and the students co-construct their learning experiences, or a low level of structure in which the students work interactively among themselves to solve problems. Will students be grouped together for the purpose of problem-solving or will the instructor teach to the whole class?

Another critical component in selecting a teaching model is to determine the type of support system that will be provided for students. Will the teacher be directive or facilitative? Will the teacher encourage productivity, independent learning, or the development of self-awareness? Will the teacher be a coach and help students learn how to work together in a group and utilize their synergy? Will the teacher be didactic, offer students feedback and encourage students to make improvements in their performance? Implementing effective learning activities requires that teachers are well-acquainted with a variety of instructional strategies and are capable of using a model that is most appropriate to the instructional purpose.

Benefits to teachers Selecting a teaching model is crucial to effective teaching. Using teaching models acknowledges that students have a variety of learning styles and thinking styles. Teaching models are selected to coincide with the learners' preferred styles of learning, the students' aptitude and the subject matter. Selecting teaching models may improve the quality of instruction because they emphasize the use of sound functional plans, and the importance of identifying clear goals for teaching.

Using a model of teaching helps teachers clarify their objectives and develop learning experiences that will help bring about successful student outcomes. Teaching models make the process of instruction more systematic because it offers a framework for guiding the processes of planning, implementation, and evaluation. In the absence of having an instructional model or a clear plan of action, teaching is a guessing game and in the worst case may become an aimless pursuit for both the student and teacher.

Teachers need a range of models to select from since there is no single model of teaching that is effective for every situation. When teachers have a variety of instructional strategies available to them, they are more able to engage students in a variety of meaningful ways that is in the best interest of learners and more closely matches the ways in which they learn best. Models help to increase the probability that certain types of learning will occur.

Benefits to students   Using teaching models benefits students by helping them: (1) increase their aptitude for learning, (2) retain information longer, (3) build their academic self-esteem, (4) learn more rapidly, and (5) facilitate different types of learning. Teaching models also acknowledge the importance of recognizing the impact of learner characteristics and aptitude on student outcomes. Models also provide a vehicle for the students to know the way in which they will be taught, what behavioral changes the instructor is trying to elicit, and gives them an opportunity to be an informed participant in their learning.

In order for learning to occur, students must often experience a feeling of disequilibrium as they begin to assimilate new knowledge into existing frameworks. "Discomfort is a precursor to growth ..." (Joyce and Weil, 1996, pp. 388–89). Selecting teaching strategies and appropriate learning activities that help students modulate their discomfort as they acquire new knowledge is an essential component of the instructor's role. Joyce and Weil (1996) claim that the way in which the learning environment is constructed also has implications for encouraging student learning.

> Properly constructed, a learning environment fits soft rather than hard metaphors. It curls around students, conforming to their characteristics just as properly treated learners also better fit soft rather than hard metaphors and can curl around the features of the learning environment (p. 392).

Teaching to Students' Learning Styles

Teachers must learn to teach differently and responsively to a wide variety of college-age students, including some individuals who may feel disenfranchised from schools or others who believe that earning a degree is an entitlement. Because students exhibit diverse learning styles, interests, talents, temperaments, and personalities, it is important that teachers present a variety of opportunities in which learning may take place.

Once the appropriate teaching model has been selected, teachers can direct their efforts towards developing learning activities that incorporate different learning styles. Learning styles represent students' consistent way of responding to and using stimuli in the context of learning. They emerge from individuals' reactions to experiences such as routines, events, and feelings (Dunn, 1996). Comprised of biologically and developmentally imposed personal characteristics, they are as individual as one's signature (Dunn, Beaudry, & Klavas, 1989). Over time, a pattern of responses or learning style tends to reoccur when one concentrates on new and difficult material.

Students usually show clear preferences or strengths in their learning styles. These learning styles exert a significant influence upon the ways in which individuals can learn. For example, some learning styles that make the same teaching method effective for some individuals render it ineffective for others. Dunn and Dunn and Price (1989) have developed a 21 element learning styles inventory. The classifications in the inventory include factors that affect students' ability to learn such as:

> (a) their immediate environment (sound, light, temperature, furniture/seating designs, (b) their own emotionality (motivation, persistence, responsibility [conformity vs. nonconformity], and need for externally imposed structure or the opportunity to do things their own way, (c) sociological preferences (learning alone, in a pair, in a small groups, as part of a team, with an authoritative or collegial adult, and wanting variety as opposed to patterns and routines), (d) psychological characteristics (perceptual strengths, time-of-day energy levels, and need for intake, mobility while learning), and (e) processing inclinations (global, analytic, right/left, and impulsive/reflective) (Dunn, 1990b, p. 225).

Knowledge of learning styles helps teachers design curriculum and learning experiences that respond to students' needs for sound level, type of illumination, temperature, seating arrangements, mobility, grouping preferences, the structure of the learning environment, and the senses (auditory, visual, verbal, or kinesthetic) through the ways in which students learn best. Dunn (1990a) also observed that students can learn almost any subject matter when they are instructed in ways that match their learning styles preferences. Because they emerge in part from biology, learning styles are remarkably resistant to change. Dunn (1990b) has reported that research

> ... has repeatedly documented that when students are taught in ways that match their preferences as measured by the Learning Style Inventory (LSI) (Dunn, Dunn, and Price, 1975, 1979, 1981, 1985, 1989), they demonstrated statistically higher achievement and attitude test scores, even on standardized tests, than when they are taught with approaches that mismatch their preferences (p.15).

Ingham (1989) observed that when adults were introduced to new material in a way that matched their perceptual preferences, they were able to recall significantly more than when introduced to material through their least preferred modality. This study underscores the importance of developing lessons that are responsive to students' various learning styles. When learning experiences coincide with students' learning styles, teachers acknowledge individual diversity and recognize that students differ in their cognitive style, conceptualizations, affect and behavior.

Cheung (1994) also reported that students learn more quickly and fully when teaching and learning activities match their learning styles. He suggested that differentiated teaching is more likely to meet the needs of heterogeneous students than a singular or fixed method of teaching. Learning styles may be reflected in learning experiences that acknowledge the different ways that people perceive and gain knowledge, form ideas and think, form values, and act.

In what ways can an awareness of students' preferred learning styles be helpful to the dance/movement therapist-teacher? Why is it important to consider learning styles when planning and teaching the curriculum? First it is important to recognize that dance/movement therapy students may differ in their learning styles dimensions. While one student may show preferences for kinesthestic learning in contrast to the auditory, visual, or cognitive domains, another might prefer learning that emphasizes the visual and auditory domains. With this knowledge in hand, the dance/movement therapist-teacher is much better positioned to teach in ways that are responsive to students' preferred learning needs. Second, it is especially important that students are challenged to acquire strengths in all domains and strengthen their abilities in areas in which they exhibit weakness so that they can work toward a balance in their awareness and facility across these domains. These skills are fundamental to practicing dance/movement therapists who must be able to keenly observe and assess clients' abilities and limitations in all of the sensory modalities. Furthermore, the therapist can use this information to create a therapeutic environment that is responsive to client's learning preferences while augmenting the clients' skills in a modality that is dysfunctional.

What sensory modalities do students use during the course of their dance/movement therapy studies? The following examples may be illustrative. Learning experiences comprised of readings, lectures, and discussion require students to use the cognitive, auditory, and visual senses. Learning experiences comprised by discussing and thinking about written material may require students to use only auditory skills. When instruction is comprised of experiential activities in which students must observe, solve problems, and reenact a therapeutic situation, they will use the visual, cognitive, and kinesthetic domains. As students learn to mirror clients' movement, they will use visual and cognitive senses. As students learn how to become attuned to clients' movements, they will use cognitive, visual, and kinesthetic sensory modalities.

In order to perceive the client's movement and communicate empathically , the therapist must be able to process information in the cognitive, visual, and kinesthetic modalities. Using this information, the therapist can mirror the client's essential movement and expressions to let him/her know that he/she was understood. The use of words as a therapeutic technique exemplifies the auditory domain. Asking clients to move using words such as: *swing, push, pull, slash,* or *punch* can encourage them to move stiffened body parts and permit the release of tension. This intervention can help clients experience catharsis or gain insight into issues that are repressed.

Developing Goals for All Students

Fostering a learning community that engages all individual learners within a classroom setting is essential for building milieus that promote learning. To create this type of environment, teachers need to realize that their classes are comprised of individual learners and be able to visualize what they want each student to acquire as a result of their instruction. Teachers must not perceive their classroom as a homogenous group of students. Planning learning experiences that are grounded in these perspectives will help teachers focus on developing a set of goals for each student. Assisting students in becoming competent and self-directed therapists necessitates that instructors are able to identify concrete goals for each student.

Teachers need to be able to construct visual as well as cognitive images of students' present ability and skill levels. They should be able to articulate an image of the skills they would like students to develop during their instruction and the methods that they would use to assist them in achieving successful outcomes. Once outcomes have been identified, teachers are better equipped to plan and sequence the types of learning activities that will be engaging and result in successful outcomes. In a pedagogical sense, this conceptualization of teaching assumes that teachers have a theoretical and practical knowledge base of the content and skills they plan to teach as well as technical expertise in instructional and evaluation methods. Teachers who have acquired this level of expertise can select from a range of instructional strategies in order to respond flexibly to learners' diverse backgrounds. For example, simply knowing how to properly organize materials can facilitate learning. If the curriculum is comprised of a wealth of didactic information, student learning can be enhanced if the instructor offers the information to students in a logical presentation format, according to principles, concepts, or facts. Using graphic organizers can also assist students (Tarleton, 1992).

Assessing students' prior knowledge, understanding how students learn and considering what motivates student learning can facilitate the instructor's ability to plan for instruction. For example, by carefully determining what students' already know the instructor is in a much better position to create learning experiences that help students understand the relevance of the material to be learned and how it is applicable. Using techniques such as brainstorming and asking students to describe what they know, what they want to know, and what they have learned (KWL) can assist with this process (Tarleton, 1992).

Demonstrating Interpersonal Skills

One of the primary tasks of teachers is to communicate, listen to and understand our students, and to speak in ways that allow us to be understood by our students. There can be no interaction between teacher and students without listening and speaking to one another or without the shared process of movement for dance therapy students. Teachers need communication and interpersonal skills that demonstrate that they are able to show respect for the dignity and humanity of each individual. They should create an environment that fosters an understanding and appreciation for different viewpoints and model an acceptance for the variety of student perspectives. The importance of demonstrating reflective listening as well as regard for the individuality of students can not be understated. Teachers should carefully consider the meanings that are embedded in students' nonverbal behavior. Students' behavioral manifestations are communications that tell us something about their experience and what's relevant in their world.

Teaching is not simply the act of telling students what to do; it is a process in which teacher and students work together for the same desired ends. Moreover, teaching requires an ability to perceive patterns, to be aware of the emergent dynamics within classrooms, to discern their meaning, and to have the ingenuity to respond in meaningful ways (Eisner, 1995). The teacher must be able to read the qualitative information that occurs in action and think on his/her feet to orchestrate the quality of instruction that respects the individual. Just as a pianist does not learn to play a concerto before learning to play scales, teachers must also acquire the rudiments of their profession. Table 3.6 depicts the characteristics of effective and ineffective teachers.

Characteristics of the Adult Learner

Who is the adult learner? What are the characteristics of their learning needs? Adult learners are generally self-directed. Often they will be mature in their attitudes, behaviors, and motivations (Westmeyer, 1988). Because they bring a rich resource of experience to the classroom, their curriculum should be built upon their need and motivation to know. Adult learners are also more motivated, task-oriented, and self-directed than pre-adult learners. The effective teacher will offer a classroom climate exemplified by mutual respect and trust, supportiveness, openness, authenticity, and pleasure. In this environment, students would be given a chance to speak and ask questions; their ideas and insights would be welcomed. Furthermore, the instructor's level of enthusiasm may catalyze student engagement so they take more pleasure in working on learning new content and undertaking new challenges. Involving students directly in decisions that can be shared will help students feel ownership for their learning and promote the feeling that the classroom milieu is theirs (Westmeyer, 1988).

TABLE 3.6 CHARACTERISTICS OF TEACHERS

	EFFECTIVE	INEFFECTIVE
Method of instruction	• Varied, matched to students' individual learning and instructors' preferred teaching style. • Helps students learn how to learn. • Modifies learning activities to accommodate individual learner needs. • Plans instruction at a variety of cognitive levels.	• Lacks a repertoire of varied instructional strategies. • Teaches students what to think. • Unaware and inattentive to students' individual learning needs and abilities. • Instruction emphasizes mechanical and rote learning.
Grouping students	Uses a variety of small and large groups and individualized activities linked to lesson plan or project outcomes.	Uses whole class instruction exclusively.
Questioning	Asks questions that require critical thinking, creativity, and synthesis.	Asks questions that necessitate yes/no responses.
Guided practice	• Provides opportunities for students to practice what they have learned. • Checks students' comprehension.	• Expects students to synthesize material on their own. • Doesn't check for students' comprehension.
Use of classroom time	Offers direct instruction, accompanied by clear expectations for instructional outcomes.	• Instruction lacks clarity, is unfocused and disorganized. • Expectations for student outcomes are unclear.
Style of interaction	• Receptive to student input and their interests. • Warm, personable, and enthusiastic. • Humane and vulnerable.	• Disinterested in subject matter and students' interests. • Cold, unengaging and unapproachable. • Directive and autocratic.
Nonverbal communication	Attentive to students' body language and facial expressions.	• Unaware and inattentive to nonverbal behaviors. • Acknowledges only verbalized communications.
Pacing	Smooth, fluid.	Dwells on irrelevant material.
Classroom milieu	• Encourages active learning. • Promotes student ownership.	• Rigid environment. • Stifles students, input and expression.
Student feedback	Offers authentic and guided feedback.	Provides inconsistent or non-evaluative feedback, or harsh criticism without ideas for improvement.

Jackson, Barnett, Caffarella, Lee and MacIsaac (1992) have emphasized that in teaching adults, instructors must consider their unique characteristics including the: (1) context of their lives, (2) role of experience and prior knowledge, and (3) differences in processes of learning. The adult learner's life is generally comprised of multiple roles and life circumstances which affect learning. Typically adults have assumed responsibility for their lives and the role of a student is an additional rather than a primary role. Exposure to life experience is one facet that differentiates the adult learner from the child learner. Adult learning tends to be motivated by a need to make sense out of life experiences and integrating, translating, and transferring new knowledge into existing schemata.

Past experiences can also be an obstacle to learning. Unlike children, adults are generally more reflective and tolerant of ambiguities and contradictions and can appreciate how disequilibrium can serve as a catalyst for developing new knowledge. Adults typically engage in identifying problems, problem-solving, and methods of inquiry. However, it is important to recognize that the construct of mental operations has a bearing on how instructors should plan for instruction. Learners who are at the level of concrete mental operations require hands-on or personal and direct experiences to make sense out of new concepts or skills. On the other hand, students who are at the formal level of operations are able to relate to new material and ideas via vicarious experiences or abstract examples (Westmeyer, 1988).

Learning in isolation has little relevance for the adult learner. In fact adults tend to learn best through experience. Instruction should not be comprised of telling students what to do. Experiential knowledge relies upon using one's own experiences along with the experiences of others to inform the process of learning. Experiential learning is best guided by constructivist teaching which assumes that learners are active participants in their construction of new knowledge. Classroom techniques that promote constructivist teaching include analysis of case studies, reflective writing, using simulations, role-playing, and asking open-ended questions. Perry (1994) suggests that open-ended questions asked in a logical sequence will challenge and motivate learners, resulting in perceptive insights.

The learning context can impact adult engagement in instruction and outcomes. Adults will respond differently to classroom experience depending on who they are as learners and how they view a specific learning activity (Jackson, Barnett, Caffarella, Lee, & MacIsaac, 1992). Teachers must be responsive to the context of learning, too. The social and cultural background of the learner and the learning situation is critical. Learners may respond differently to learning activities depending on who they are as learners and how they perceive an activity. Learners may feel competent and comfortable to engage and share in new learning situations or they may be uncomfortable and even hostile. How the teacher responds to the context of the learner can impact the perceptions about his/her demeanor and approachability for the entire milieu.

Effective teachers adjust their instruction to complement students' experiences, offer feedback that is relevant to their developmental level, and create learning environments that are less controlling and structured (Bohlin, Milheim, & Viechnicki, 1993–1994). Ultimately one goal of effective instruction is to empower adult learners and strengthen their confidence as critical thinkers. By showing students that their abilities are adequate and trustworthy, their critical confidence becomes strengthened and their capacity to exercise critical thinking becomes enhanced (Boerckel & Barnes, 1991).

Bohlin, Milheim, and Viechnicki (1993–1994) have offered several strategies to make instruction more appealing. They suggest that the instruction can stimulate greater student interest and improve the students' effort if the instructor: (1) models enthusiasm and captures the interest of the learner, (2) increases the learner's curiosity by presenting challenging problems, (3) demonstrates the relevance of instruction, (4) allows flexibility in course assignments so that the learner's personal goals can be met, (5) promotes the learner's confidence, (6) clearly states course requirements to improve the learner's expectancy for success, and (7) provides regular and immediate feedback so that the learner can be apprised of his/her progress. Using variety in the presentation of content can also stimulate increased student engagement in learning (Perry, 1994). In order to improve the instructional effort of adult learners the instructor should: (1) improve the learners' confidence by gradually increasing the level of difficulty in instructional activities, (2) provide assignments that allow learners to apply material in practical situations, (3) give supportive feedback to increase learners' confidence, (4) relate material to be learned to real life situations, and (5) provide feedback that links the learners' success or failure to their level of effort and ability.

Field experiences are an integral component to students' curricular experiences. Performed at a practice site under the mentorship of current practitioners or with clinically trained instructors, these experiences should be designed to:

1. help students synthesize classroom teaching with actual practice.

2. afford students an opportunity to develop an individualized plan of study.

3. include a seminar so that instructors can encourage students to reflect upon field experiences, and students and instructors can solve field-based problems.

4. provide mentorship and introduction into professional roles.

Richey (1992) stated that learning is phenomenologically and contextually bound. He discriminated between models of learning and actual processes of learning. Although cognitive models of the process of learning are mechanical, the actual processes are experiential. He also suggested that when adults enjoy their learning experiences, they are more likely to transfer newly acquired knowledge to their jobs. In order to promote the transfer of learning, he suggests that instructors: (1) teach foundational information in a meaningful way and demonstrate its relevance to practice-based situations, (2) offer students an opportunity to apply conceptual knowledge in a variety of situations, (3) emphasize students' use of inductive thinking, and (4) promote the use of metacognitive strategies.

Understanding who the adult learner is in relationship to the style of field-dependence/independence and its implication for self-directed learning or the need for a supportive interpersonal learning environment is crucial (Joughin, 1992). Witkin, Moore, Goodenough, and Cox (1977) defined field-dependence/independence as

> the extent to which the person perceives part of a field as discrete from the surrounding field as a whole, rather than embedded in the field; or the extent to which the organization of the prevailing field determines the perception of its components; or to put it in everyday terminology, the extent to which the person perceives analytically (pp. 6, 7).

The field dependent individual is likely to experience difficulty solving problems ". . . where the solution involves taking some critical element out of the context in which it was presented and restructuring the problem material so that the item is now used in a different context" (Witkin, et al., 1977, p. 8).

Joughin (1992) has suggested that field-dependent/independent learners respond in significantly different ways to key elements in learning situations such as structure, analytical ability, response to affective considerations, and authority/responsibility. Adult learners are likely to respond according to their need for external structure, will show marked difference in their ability to master situations that call for a high level of analytic ability, vary in their need for supportive environments, and are likely to show varying responses to authority. Witkin et al. (1977) described several of the educational implications of field dependent learners.

1. They tend to learn social material better than field independent learners.
2. They tend to require externally defined goals and reinforcements; field independent learners tend to have self-defined goals and reinforcements.
3. In contrast to field independent learners, they have difficulty in unstructured learning situations or coping with material that is disorganized. They need more explicit instruction in problem solving.
4. They favor instruction that allows for interaction.

Even (1982) has observed that field dependent students do not work well independently, do not learn from lectures, and have a strong need for discussion, small group work, and outlines. In contrast, field independent learners prefer to work alone, learn well from lectures and prefer to avoid working in small groups. Field dependent learners prefer teachers who are warm, friendly, supportive, and organized, while field independent learners are relatively unaffected by the teacher's demeanor. Field independent learners tend to be much more self-directed than field dependent learners.

By understanding the nature of adult learners, teachers are in a much better position to discriminate between relevant and irrelevant student experiences. Recognizing students' construct of mental operations and cognitive style can also help teachers plan experiences that are accessible to students.

Characteristics of the Dance/Movement Therapy Student

Who is the dance/movement therapy student? What type of individuals gravitate towards this profession? Typically students tend to be a mixture of both field-dependent and field-independent learners. Aspiring dance/movement therapists may also be dancers who seek to apply their training and background to therapeutic fields or therapists who have some background in dance and plan to expand their application of dance therapeutically. It is crucial that future dance/movement therapists have solid training in dance, so that they have a repertoire of movement as well as feelings about movement. Many of the students we interviewed shared that the love for dance and an interest in working with people propelled them towards the profession. A student from China shared that she "liked to work with people" and do body work. She also shared that she "loved to dance since she was a child." When she went to Columbia College, she checked out a college catalogue and discovered the dance/movement therapy program. After meeting with Ganet-Sigel for 30 minutes, she decided to become a dance/movement therapist.

Other students recounted how life experiences influenced their desire to become a dance/movement therapist. One student reported that "[I] started off doing modern dance" and "had experiences that opened me up to possibilities of using movement therapeutically. I didn't just realize how movement could be therapeutic, I experienced it . . . some personal revelations made me think maybe dance/movement therapy was something to go into."

Another student discussed the therapeutic benefits of dance and shared that:

> Dancing kept me sane throughout my life, healed me and expressed my pains and joy. Dance gave me a place to release feelings. In undergraduate social work program, [I] took theater movement classes and saw the power of nonverbal communication. [I] met with a co-worker who told me about D/MT after I realized my desire to incorporate more movement into working with kids and teens.

Other students sought to blend the role of dance/movement with other roles. One student shared that she was: ". . . pulled toward both art of dance and wanting to work with people. [I had] heard of D/MT through a friend. [This] seemed to be very logical for me to put the two together from the two pulls I felt."

One individual who is now a practicing psychodramatist explained how she had been

> . . . exposed to D/MT and psychodrama. Someone suggested to me that since I needed a masters to become certified as a psychodramatist, why didn't I get it in D/MT. [I] saw how effective D/MT and psychodrama was with students and my intention was to blend D/MT with psychodrama.

Another student felt that a background in dance/movement therapy was essential to her role as a dance teacher. She shared that: "In therapy training, I would gain access to interiority. There's a lot of background information on the teaching-learning process and processes in therapy that help dance teachers better understand delving into very deep places in the inner being."

In order to be accepted into the program, students are assessed to determine how much they're in touch with their bodies, what kind of training they have for physical awareness, and how well they move. Faculty members conduct observations to determine if prospective students lack a relationship to their body completely, have any consciousness, as well as any connection between their mind and their body. Efforts are also made to discern if they're moving authentically, and have an interiority. Faculty members observe students and look to see whether they have a capacity of flexibility, tempo, dynamics, meter, and rhythm and whether they're kinetically connected. If movement is inauthentic and they are asked to strike or punch, but they lack energy behind it, then questions are raised about their awareness of their own body. Movement assessments are conducted to see if students have a connection between their inner body and outer space.

Prospective students participate in a two part group movement assessment workshop after they have completed a written application. In the first part, they participate in modern dance technique activity. As applicants move, the admission's committee assesses their ability to move. For example as they sit on the floor, the faculty determines if they have an awareness of their spine, and how they use their abdominal muscles. Faculty will also try to ascertain if prospective students have the ability to move their scapula, have a good anatomical sense of their bodies, or a sense of their inner bodies. During standing exercises, students are assessed to determine if they: (1) have any capacity to use their weight in a movement sense, (2) are aware of the functioning of their hamstring muscles and their abductors, (3) can use their central channels on top of their legs, (4) can connect their chi to their legs, (5) are connected to the base, (6) have a connection to all things in space, (7) can move their spine or drop their weight well, and (8) are able to adjust their four-legged animal to a two-legged animal position in a manner that does not stress their body. Students are also asked to move across the floor to demonstrate if they know how to impulse their bodies.

In the second portion of the movement assessment, prospective students participate in a group dance/movement therapy session. During this activity, dance/movement faculty assess the applicants' awareness and expression of creativity in the absence of someone guiding their movement. They also assess how applicants move through movement words that reflect self-esteem, and how they show joy, anger, or aggression. Faculty assess the applicants' capacity for moving authentically and observe how they relate to others in the group. Faculty also observe students to determine if they know how to move through space and with inner excitement. The students' ability to just be inside of themselves, to relate to others, to relate to space, to be able to do things like punch, fall, rise, roll, move in other senses rather than the more specific senses are also assessed.

Ganet-Sigel as Dance/Movement Therapist-Teacher

Jane Ganet-Sigel uses a variety of learning experiences to offer students a very eclectic approach to learning. She incorporates simulations, role-playing, didactic teaching, inquiry training, and inductive thinking in her teaching. These activities emphasize learning through a variety of sensory modalities. While some learning experiences may only necessitate skills in one modality, at other times, students will need to use a combination of skills in the kinesthetic, visual, auditory, and/or cognitive modalities. Guest speakers are also frequently invited to offer a variety of perspectives, not all of which Ganet-Sigel personally ascribes to in her own clinical practice. In her dance/movement theory classes, students are responsible for their own learning and are given opportunities to lead groups. For example, to fulfill a course requirement, they present a theoretical approach from concept to actual practice. First, they are expected to give a report and handouts of information they have researched. Next, they apply conceptual knowledge to the group and take the role of the therapist in a simulated therapeutic process as the other students assume the role of patients. The goal of simulations is to approximate realistic conditions in clinical practice. The problem-solving activities and the concepts learned are applicable to understanding and performing relevant tasks in actual therapeutic interventions. As they apply theoretical approach/technique to the class "group," Ganet-Sigel critiques their work. One student described the impact of this process.

> The way we learned how to be therapists really was, in a way, through practicing on ourselves. So there was all this ripe material of our own issues coming up. So it was hard sometimes to make the difference or to find a difference between your own issues, put that aside, and to learn what you were there to learn. It could become mixed up. Jane was there to kind of help you separate that. And in the end, I found that very valuable.

Students often reported feeling excited about applying the technique of a theorist, but they soon realized that they had to be sensitive and responsive to the dynamic and context of the group session itself. As one student confessed:

> I would walk out of class thinking "Oh, this is really neat. I want to try this," but I was also very aware when I went into group that I wasn't going to be able to try something out unless it fit with what was happening.

Ganet-Sigel urges students to apply what they have learned into practice rather than focus on what grades they earn in the course. While students are challenged to achieve perfection, they quickly learn that there is no cookbook approach. Instead they must learn to demonstrate an ability to use the techniques or the material. According to one student: "she emphasized how you put what you learned into practice, how deep it went inside you rather than grades."

Students have ample opportunity to practice what they learned. During three internship placements they learn to become astute observers by offering detailed reports about how they saw clients move. This activity serves two purposes. First, it helps students demonstrate their understanding of the connections between theory and practice. Second, it permits Ganet-Sigel to check in with students and to see what they have understood.

Later in the internship, she coaches students on becoming attuned with their clients. She often tells students that "things will come up from the client; our job is to just be there and give them space." She will correct students' actions when it has become apparent that their actions resulted from their own ego rather than arising from the clients' needs. As one student observed,

> I think that a lot of us are unaware of what's going on within us and have a great desire to fix people. And I think one of the things that she would do is to get us away from that. So a lot of times, people would take the theories and say, okay, well, I'm going to use this theory on this person and that will fix them. And I think in the times that she would correct us were times we were coming from that place of not really being where the clients were at, but coming from our own need to fix people. And one thing I remember her saying a lot was, less is more.

She would say, "Stop directing and start watching what's already happening." And I remember her coming to one of my sessions, when she came to observe me in my internship, I was just shouting out directions to the group. She told me to "Just shut up and start listening to what's going on."

She encourages students to probe into things that they have read and be reflective about their experiences. She also urges them to find out about themselves in the process of becoming a therapist and discover their own way in understanding how different approaches can be used in clinical practice. To facilitate this process, students maintain a journal and write about the experiences that they have had during simulated groups.

Through telling stories, Ganet-Sigel helps exemplify what she's teaching. For example, she provides a bridge between content and clinical practice by giving students a historical account of her work as a dance/movement therapist, sharing anecdotes from her practice, and then opening up her presentation for discussion. Students reported that ". . . when she spoke about her own history as a dance/movement therapist, that this was important. But it was also equally important . . . the way she had other means of presenting the material." Ganet-Sigel is also attuned to the different ways that students learn best. Rather than relying solely on the auditory mode of presentation, she also recognizes the importance of visual tools. She uses videotapes of her own work in various therapeutic settings to acknowledge students' particular learning needs and how they are able to receive communication.

In the group dynamics course, she tends to be more didactic in her teaching style. In this course, students learn about a variety of approaches to group therapy and some basic principles regarding the therapist's role and techniques with groups. As one student stated, "she had the flexibility to know when to be directional and didactic and when to urge that more come from the students themselves." In this class, students are asked to take certain concepts and apply them to an actual situation in a take-home exam. For example, they were asked to compare a variety of methods effecting change through the group process. Table 3.7 presents some of the questions that students were asked to answer.

Following this exam, one student commented that:

> . . . I felt excited that I had had a chance to pull together all [the] information we'd talked about for 7 1/2 weeks. [It] felt good to be responsible for and participate actively in one's own learning. Jane had the facility to go back and forth between different instructional styles [which was very helpful to me]. She held high expectations for her class.

An Analysis of Ganet-Sigel's Models of Teaching

Depending upon the nature of the course she teaches and the experiences she plans for students, Ganet-Sigel uses a variety of teaching models. While teaching courses in dance/movement therapy theory she engages in co-constructing curriculum and invites them to take a leadership role. They become active learners and offer interpretations and ideas about the ways that theoretical approaches can be applied to the practice of dance/movement. Rather than simply accepting Ganet-

Table 3.7   FINAL EXAMINATION FOR GROUP DYNAMICS (METHODS OF GROUP THERAPY)

Directions: Answer three of the remaining questions that you did not answer on your mid-term exam in an essay format.

I.
1. Yalom talks about eleven (11) curative factors (page 71). Expand on any five (5) factors of your choice—plus group cohesiveness.
2. What is meant by interpersonal learning as a mediation of change?
3. What is meant by The Group as a Social Microcosm?
4a). What are some determinants of Group Cohesiveness?
4b). What are the sources of high and low cohesiveness?
5. What are some basic tasks of the therapist and some of the roles that the therapist plays in the therapy group situation?
6. What are some of the criteria for excluding and including patients in a therapy group?
7. What are some methods of composing a therapy group? Some considerations as to place/time/size/preparation of the group?

II. Describe common issues to all types of groups
1. when a group is just beginning.
2. when a group has been going for some time (an advanced group).
3. typical problem patients and how they affect a group.

III. Describe the difference in the formats and procedures in conducting any five (5) of the following groups:

1. Self Help Groups
2. Psychoanalytic Groups
3. Family Therapy Groups
4. Encounter Groups
5. Gestalt Groups
6. Art Therapy Groups
7. Dance/movement therapy Groups
8. Groups with Co-Therapists
9. Psycho-drama Groups
10. T-Groups
11. Alcoholic & Drug Groups
12. Adolescent Groups
13. Children's Groups

IV. Elaborate on your preferences of the type of group you would prefer to lead. Why? What attributes and knowledge do you have for such a group?

V. Extra Question: What are the pros and cons of individual versus group therapy, the advantages, and disadvantages of a combination of individual and group therapy for one patient?

Sigel's viewpoint or one viewpoint about theory, her students analyze, critique, and share their findings.

Experiential activities serve as a core of her instruction. Students actually move concepts. As one former student observed, "you have to move it to learn it. Ganet-Sigel encouraged us to make the behavior she wanted us to learn our own and practice it." Another former student shared that

> Jane is responsible for the fact that I think that students at Columbia, more than probably any other program, have a very diverse clinical background when they finish. She makes sure that you get into a lot of different situations where you get experience with different populations, so you have a lot of clinical experience when you're finished.

Role playing and simulation are employed to help students assimilate and apply the techniques of dance/movement therapy. In other circumstances such as the group dynamics course, she is relatively more didactic in her approach. In this course, she focuses on helping students acquire new concepts and build a knowledge base in dance/movement therapy. During the final examination, inquiry training is used to help students synthesize their knowledge and apply it in relevant situations.

There is little doubt that one of her major goals is to help students become the best therapists possible. She serves as a strong mentor and guide in the development of aspiring therapists. This point was aptly illustrated by one student who commented:

> I think when Jane knew that you really wanted to become a dance therapist and that you wanted to work really hard, she showed a great faith. She always said, "There's no right way. There's no wrong way. It's only your way." And even though she had strong opinions of what it is to be a therapist and she practiced her own way, if you found your own way and it was organic to you, she respected it. Even if she maybe didn't agree with it. I think that was what she was interested in.

Another student described Ganet-Sigel's capacity for mentoring.

> Jane has been really like a rock for people. That's how I could really describe her, like a rock. Because she stays in the center of what dance therapy is. And so you can always touch base with the rock. I don't know what will happen when she stops doing her work. There's just nobody that could replace her. For the students, she can be very intimidating . . . But . . . they learn over time that her strengths, even though she can be intimidating, is something that they need to have and [need] to have modeled. Because when they get out into the world, they need that same kind of strength to deal with a lot of misconceptions about dance therapy and the prejudice in the psychiatric hospitals and in the medical community. And . . . so [since] they've had that modeling from her . . . they can draw upon that . . .
> . . . there's a lot of crumbling that takes place in the training because students are doing these exercises, [that are] very powerful, [with] all this stuff is coming up, they should be in therapy. Not all of them are. [But] even for those [who] are, it's almost not

enough because we can't do therapy in class or really complete some of these things to the point where healing in the student would take place . . . so they go through this crumbling process of their false stuff, and in the process there's a lot of transference on the teachers and especially on Jane.

[Since] Jane serves as a rock, [who] can be intimidating, students sometimes experience an increased sense of anxiety. And they go through a period of time where they're mad at her, and they don't understand why she's the way she is. . . . [But] then when they graduate, they're all so grateful. It's like, wow, they learned what that was all about. They're out in the world. They're facing a lot of important things. And she was always there like a rock. And she still would be. Anytime a student calls her, an alumni, a colleague, she is right there with help. She backs you up. She backs you up with letters if [you are] a non-registered dance therapist or [if an] untrained one would come in and try to take your job. She backs you up in every way possible professionally. So she's very committed, very strong in that way, and very helpful.

One other former student, and a colleague communicated quite eloquently the role changes that the teacher and student experience through the process of mentoring. She described how Ganet-Sigel facilitated her growth as a professional and accommodated her changes during this delicate process.

[I] guess I could just say my relationship went through many transitions where I started out as a student and ended up [becoming] a colleague and very good friend . . . one of the things that I really value in my relationship with Jane is that she has been able to accommodate all those changes that we've gone through. I really feel at this point that there's a real receptivity to me and my input. It's like . . . at this end point, our roles are beginning to reverse. Just beginning, as she enters into her seventies and is moving towards retirement. I can just feel the beginning of that. She's been my mentor all these years. And it's not that I'm going to become her mentor or anything, but that there is that development of . . . no longer being the child or, the student . . . and that she fully accepts me as her equal.

I want to comment on her ability to adapt and to be flexible to facilitate that. I feel like there's this real mutual respect . . . so I can feel in myself that I've really moved from being the scared admiring student to still be admiring but admiring from a different stance. These comments aptly illustrate a point when the mentoree . . . grows up and becomes an equal . . . even in the midst of standing side by side and feeling an equality, [I feel] an increased admiration . . . as I look back and kind of see all of that and see how her love of dance therapy and her openness to creating growth in that field has also created growth for many individuals . . . .

She seeks to help students develop their capacity for leadership, too. She acknowledges students and encourages authentic communication without reprisal for their candor. One student recounted an incident in which she fought with her and ended up yelling at her.

> She was picking on me about how I was skipping and I just got so angry and I just yelled at her — I just yelled, "I know how to fucking skip!" And she just said, "Oh, I see you do." I felt like it was a test. And she was so strong, and I felt like she wanted to know what we were made of.

Another student shared that "I always felt that Jane had a faith in me, and that really helped me get through the program."

One former student recalled an in-class experience when Ganet-Sigel called upon her to assume a leadership role during a simulated dance/movement group therapy session.

> . . . there have been a few times when I felt criticized, but . . . I do remember my initial leadership experience. And it was painful, not because of the critique, but just because. . . . I remember doing psychotics, and I just remember my sense of helplessness that there was so much going on in the room, and so I remember that experience kind of fondly but — I remember Jane sort of laughing with me at the helplessness, but the class really, they loved to get on and do these character role things. They were being atrociously psychotic.

Many students observed that Ganet-Sigel wasn't afraid of things that were uncomfortable. The behavior she demonstrated was described by another student as

> . . . it was like there was no fear. In her body and actions she said to students, "Let's go after this and let's learn it." [This form of teaching actually] became positive [method] for me. She helped me really appreciate that when you're a therapist, you're working with people and their most private, special, hurtful, angry emotions. And you have to be ready for that, to honor and pay homage to your patients.

Another student commented:

> I liked Jane. I loved her as a teacher and as a friend. It could be difficult on me, and I can remember yelling back at her, but that kind of made it more rich for me. She was a real person that you could bounce off against. She wasn't fake. I think that's very refreshing to find someone who's so real.

Ganet-Sigel had little interest in cultivating merely technicians.

> She would talk about your need to have it all at your fingertips, but go into a session being completely open to what is happening there and responding to that. Everything's done with the gloves

off. Look you're not going to be a good therapist if you don't look at this, deal with that, or get this information straight, 'cause I don't think you're using it maximally here.

[Or she would say] . . . you have all this other pile of information and all those things that we had talked about, and I didn't see you apply that in this simulated session, and it seems to me like you're — it was set up. In the simulation, that would have been an obvious body of knowledge to draw on. And you made some therapeutic choices there in this simulated session, that were okay, but did you give any thought or consideration to this possibility?

Ganet-Sigel was remembered by many of her students for saying, "I don't want to turn out dance therapists. I want to turn out damn good dance therapists." Concurring with this point of view, another former student reported that "Jane made every effort to help all students deserve their diplomas, and to be the best dance/movement therapists in the Chicago area." One student recounted that

. . . she would be disappointed in us when we hadn't done something well. And when Jane was disappointed, she could seem quite sharp. And so, that was a little bit challenging for me, and I know for other people as well. And I think where it became the most complicated [when] at one point she was the only person doing dance movement therapy in Chicago.

Experiencing disequilibrium is often a precursor to learning as one student observed.

Learning occurs when you're in a place that's uncomfortable, usually. And that's why I think that Jane was a good teacher. I was uncomfortable a lot because I was at the edge of my knowledge. She knew stuff I didn't know, and she gave that information very generously. But sometimes when the information comes out, you know, it stings, because you feel like you should have known it.

Ganet-Sigel deeply influenced one woman who later became a psychodramatist.

I realized that there's an analogy to having been raised Catholic. I can't get away from it, even though I don't practice it. It's hard to erase. You see, I don't think of myself as dance movement therapist. I think of myself as a creative arts therapist. However, my work is informed by dance movement therapy and it's somatically based. When I'm working with clients, I always ask myself, "How is this person living within his/her body? How is this person moving within space? And how is this person using his/her body?" In drama therapy, there are two schools of theoretical thought. One is the developmental approach, and one is the role theory approach. And I guess that I come at it from a role theory approach and I think of what Moreno, the founder of psychodrama, says: We find out who we are by trying out new roles. It's the client's movement repertoire that informs me about their body. And as a therapist, I use the concept of "bodies" in more ways than just movement, and this allows me to consider more than just movement, for example, voice. But by focusing on movement, it is sort of foundational to my understanding the client. So the analogy is that I was raised as a dance movement therapist by mother Jane.

How did students respond to Ganet-Sigel's approach to teaching? Students concurred that she was a tough instructor and had a no-nonsense approach to her teaching. She could be very blunt and direct. This often facilitated student learning. As one student shared,

> it helped me learn a whole lot in a short amount of time. . . . Although you might not want to hear [it at the time], there have been times when she had said something that sounded really right to me. But I think it has been helpful for me; I've grown to really appreciate Jane a whole lot . . . Some of her criticisms have helped me grow as a therapist. . . .

Ganet-Sigel carefully modeled for students the kind of strength that they would need to manifest as they entered the world as practitioners, as observed by the following students.

> There were times she could be tough, but, it was . . . okay. Because, that was supported by concern for the individual as well as concern for what she was doing. I guess when I say tough, [I mean that] she kind of drove through the trees, you couldn't muck around. She just kind of went for it. I think one of the first classes I had with her, it was really funny, because . . . she did this little exercise where you were supposed to set up your space. And then she divided us into half, I'm sure you've done this, and one half was supposed to set up their space and then the other group was supposed to move into the space. And I was paired off with this guy that was very meek and mild.
>
> He [would come] up to my space and . . . he really did not invade it, . . . it was like home. And so, I felt fine, I sat there with him and we're just kind of playing while everybody else was fighting. And I recall that she said as we were reflecting on it, "Well, you were really a very mild kind of thing." And I was like, Well, I'm a mild kind of person. And she said, "Okay. let's do this again." And so I set up my space, and she came in [pushing] like gangbusters. And it was major, major fighting. And [she was really showing me that] "Sure you are this mild person, but you also have this other dimension, and this was what I was trying to get at."

Another student shared that although Ganet-Sigel pushed students hard, this was not problematic during her experience.

> During my internship I had terrible difficulty with the group I was working with on the day that Jane came to observe me. The whole group just fell apart. She stopped me right away and gave me very tough criticism. She said, "What's your problem?" I answered that I was losing control. She retorted: "It's not that you are losing control, you're just controlling. You're putting your head into their heads." Well I thought I was going to lose control.
>
> Then she told me I was too controlling and directed me to re-do the group. And she said, "I'm here to be your teacher, not your therapist. I'm not here to care for your emotional problems. You need to know how to take care of yourself. I'm here to be your teacher." Actually I liked that. Some teachers confuse the therapist's role and the teacher's role. Jane didn't.

This student found Jane's difficult feedback helped her grow as a therapist. She stated that:

> Jane was just so honest, black and white. When you are wrong, you are just wrong. No matter how much she likes you, you're wrong.

Another student confessed that "one night before I did group the first time I wrote an outline to help me guide the group's movement activities. I asked Ganet-Sigel about what I should do. She said, "Never do that." She told the student that she would have to train herself to feel the clients right away. "Then your techniques automatically come from your own viscera." This is one of the fundamental concepts that she imparts to students. Ganet-Sigel told the student that:

> Until you know that, I am not going to tell you too much about techniques because you're not ready. You simply want to apply those techniques to a patient and that's not right. In so many cases, you don't know what's going to happen, you can never have enough techniques for all kinds of cases. You must observe, listen, and feel your client, then you will come to discover what techniques to use.

Another student talked about how Ganet-Sigel pushed students to their fullest potential.

> [Jane] talked a lot about your growing edge, your level of tolerance for something, like loud noise — and you could only stand it so long before you went over the edge. I felt Jane took me to my growing edge — not always enjoyable; extremely valuable. She did that by being direct and frank. She wasn't afraid of things that were uncomfortable.
>
> [She has an] incredible quality of honesty and directness. Therapy confronted me with issues about myself. [I] learned some things about myself, a great gift. [She] doesn't patronize or coddle. [She] is an authentic communicator, direct teacher, and facilitator for students to learn processes. [She] taught students to use clients' agendas, not their own. She directed her energies toward making students be the best they could be by driving them and pushing

them to their limits. She demands that they move out of themselves, move out of their preconceived notions and agendas, and learn to empathize and hear with their third or second ear and their second body what's really happening with the client. [Students would] have to learn [how] to be a rock for their clients. They could not be wishy-washy or let their clients get into their boundaries and stuff.

One long time friend concurred with students' sentiments:

I think she is wonderful at allowing her students and the people who know her to not only love her, but honor her. There are some teachers who are respected and loved and all that but who don't elicit the kind of affectionate regard and attachment that she does. I think there's something about her that is open to having the students and friends say, well come over to my country and lecture. She handles that very, very well. I mean, like a real worldly sophisticate. I know what it's like to be in a different culture and talk about things that they don't know much about. She does it with great ease, and I'm sure she's not exaggerating when she explains how heartily she was welcomed and how grateful they were for what she was doing.

How did students respond to the demands of this instructor? One student shared that at times, she "felt nervous or afraid." On the other hand, she said:

[I] really admired and respected her; and felt she wanted the best for me. Jane was strong enough to make a space for me to do that hard work. She emphasized the reality that you have to come face to face with yourself if you want to be a good therapist. You have to be honest with yourself. Her faith in me never wavered and I could feel how she supported my work. Just how much dance/movement therapy meant to her inspired me. She really knows how to help you find your way.

Another student admitted: "getting so mad, [that I would want to] kick her butt. [She] gave me stuff to work on about my responses to an authority figure. [This raised] the full range of who I am as a learner."
Another student revealed that:

I think Jane was disappointed because I wasn't actually a dancer. She'd often use me as an example of less graceful movements. I didn't have the nerve to tell her how much that hurt me. She had ability to seem quite critical. I had the capacity to take it internally and hoard bad feelings. Sometimes it felt awkward between the two of us. She had a difficult time appreciating my desire to marry dance with drama. She'd remind me that we weren't here to be creative arts therapists who just dabble, that we were dance/movement therapists. She was a PURIST. It dismayed her that I wasn't; it dismayed me that she couldn't accept it because Chace used drama therapy. We had some "clearing" sessions as I went through the program. We'd re-establish the emotional connection and I'd

fail to talk about my discomfort about being pointed out as someone who was less than graceful. She had a *hard* edge. She's determined and opinionated, but her heart's in the right place. I was
angry, I chose to reframe it so as I supervise, I can critique gra-
ciously, because of what I learned from her when it wasn't given gra-
ciously. I felt angry when I felt she was thoughtless, but I had so
much respect for what she was doing . . . [I felt that] . . . she taught
[with] so much genuine caring. My primary felt emotion was love.

Another student reported that she felt

encouraged, supported, [and] frustrated. [I] wanted more techniques [and] would have preferred at times that she would present
theories and not let students run the course. [However,] I like the
idea of giving us an experience of leading. . . . [Overall] I felt I got
the kind of tools that I really wanted to get.

Another student reported feeling a little tense and nervous.

During my first field placement with her as supervisor, I was just
shaking. However I quickly learned that if you speak up for yourself, she helps you. I asked her to show me how to do it and she
did. If you're honest with her, tell her what you feel and need,
she'll let you do it. She tries to get students to show her what they
are capable of doing. She's very straight as a teacher. If you have a
complaint, talk it over with her. She'll be fine.

She's really very honest and you can be honest with her. You
don't have to torture yourself. I appreciated her criticism. I learned
a lot from it. I love her. She has such affection. She has such a felt
power from her body; students are attracted to her. If you are
doing well, she gives students great compliments and recommendations. She is anxious to see her students become good
dance/movement therapists. She really prepares students to go out
and become good dance/movement therapists. For example, she
gave me the kind of encouragement that enhanced my self-esteem.
I was proud to be her student. Overall you can feel love from her.

How does Ganet-Sigel help students connect theory into practice?
One student replied that she makes

you come face to face with yourself [and] makes you learn it your
own [way]. [She helps] you to dig as deep down inside . . . by
doing . . . by confronting you. The way we learned how to be
therapists was really in a way practicing on ourselves.

Others shared that "she insisted that students learn to stay in the present and respond to what's going on with the client. Although feedback
during practice sessions could be positive, it didn't always feel positive
at the time to some students." However as one student observed,
"Some things I heard about my style have stayed with me; that's a positive learning experience."

A painful lesson about the pitfalls of countertransference was remembered by another former student.

> I was in my field placement working with psychotic children, and Jane was my supervisor; it was my first day. And this is how I learned about countertransference. In the room came a little girl in a pink party dress, really adorable little girl and I thought, "Why is she even in here? She's so cute." And she held my hand, and I could feel nothing. I felt no energy coming from her. And I looked at her again, and I realized that she really had had no mothering. And I started to cry. And Jane took one look at me and said, "Who's the patient here, you or her?" That was it. That was the end of countertransference for me, and this helped me keep my boundaries.

Another student reported that

> [She] led us to open our minds, to understand our own body and listen to ourselves from our center. The way you learn everything, you have to observe, you have to be there, non-judgmentally. Use your own mirroring techniques. With hospital patients, my body reacts to them; I don't talk too much. They can feel your face, your whole body, your whole energy. They trust you. They feel that you're there with them and like "Yeah, I know you really care for us."

Another student expressed with excitement her dedication and willingness to supervise her field experience.

> She made it possible for me to do the program. [She] drove from Chicago to Milwaukee to provide supervision. In fact [she] drove everywhere to visit students on days she wasn't teaching. [She] collected faculty who were willing to go way beyond what they were paid to do and put in a lot more hours than their paycheck would indicate. All of them had this marvelous directness and presence to observing how you were learning.

Moreover, the program "attracted fantastic students who were extraordinary human beings."

Ganet-Sigel also taught students about the importance of being attuned with the clients' developmental readiness rather than being punitive to clients who weren't ready for the group process. During a meeting with an intern, they talked about working with inpatients and the hospital's policy of sending a nonparticipating client back to his/her room. Suggesting another approach to this situation, she told the student that he/she have could have the client simply sit on the edge of the room and return to the group at some point and invite him/her to return to the circle when they were comfortable. In this way, she sensitized the future therapist to both patient's needs as well as the politics of the environment or institution where he/she might later become employed.

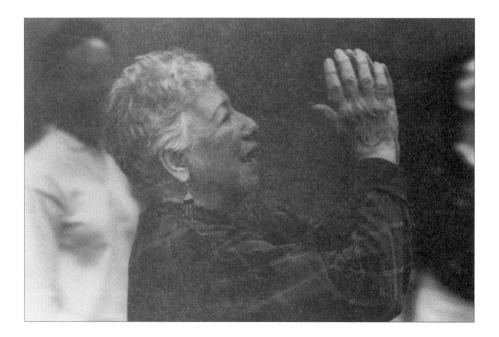

One of her former students, now a colleague, also described how Ganet-Sigel teaches students to become therapists.

> I think that one of the major things that she teaches is she tries to get students to get themselves out of the way of the process. And by that, I mean to facilitate in a way that you don't interfere, that you give very simple structure, that you find out where your clients are at, and that you don't impose an agenda on that. And so that you make room for whatever needs to happen to happen. And that sounds very easy, but that really means that you have to have a handle on your own stuff. . . . She allows for a lot of creativity . . . she really wants you to be creative, but that in being creative, you have to be creative in a way that you don't get in the way of what needs to happen. So that's no mean task.

This individual, a former student and now a colleague spoke of the challenges associated with this approach.

> Sometimes there are some struggles around that. One of the many things she said to our faculty is that we can't try to teach these students everything we've learned through our years of experience. And so even in that there's a statement of allowing the student to struggle with where they're at.

Ganet-Sigel places the onus for learning on the students' shoulders in part by encouraging them to synthesize their own learning. In effect, she is committed to teaching students a process, but some students enter the program with an expectation that they are simply going to be given techniques and skills or learn a "how to" approach to becoming a therapist. Although students may come into the program want-

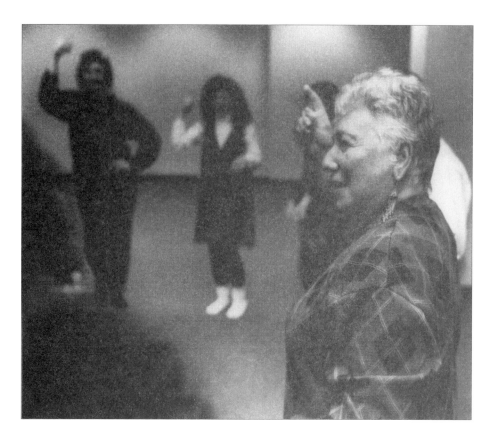

ing to just learn procedures, Ganet-Sigel remains focused on teaching the process. Concurring, one student remarked, "I guess it's one of the feelings that I still experience today . . . [her emphasis on the] process."

She takes her students on a journey as they learn to feel and understand the process of becoming a therapist. In many ways, they must trust her and be willing to travel together so that they can experience and feel what dance therapy is about. As students journey with Ganet-Sigel, what kind of transformation might they experience? In what ways do they experience changes, and how does it occur? One her former students shared that:

> Well certainly it's a slow transition. And I guess that's why it's hard to put it into words. 'Cause it happens over time. A phrase that I found myself using at times, kind of jokingly, is, "I feel right now that I could make a rock move if I had to. I could facilitate movement from a rock. . . ."
>
> . . . one of the main strategies — well, strategy, technique, approaches — that we learn as dance therapists is to attune to the other, through our bodies, through our verbal expressions, whatever. And so that as you learn to attune, a lot of things happen. You are learning to be in the moment. And this attunement is akin to Marian Chace's original mirroring. So in the fullest sense of that, you're attuning. . . .

> Stern breaks attuning down into essentially space, time, and force terms, which are terms we use in dance therapy. So it's really about being with someone in the moment. So you're really in the moment, you're really living with someone. And then besides attuning and being with someone, you're using your empathic powers to try to understand at the same time. So in a sense, in a bodily sense, you're attuning to space, time, and force. In the emotional sense, you're putting yourself in the other person's world.

Students learn how to feel what clients are feeling in their world.

> . . . In the body — in the movement sense. You're observing the timing, the rhythm of their movement. You're observing the spatial aspects. You're observing the dynamic intensity factors. Energy level. And you're attuning — you might not be attuning to all of that at the same time, and it's actually not necessary for an experience of attuning for you to be at all those modes at once, but you could be — and at the same time as you're experiencing that in your body, you're also using . . . your psyche, your emotions, your cognitive powers to, to imagine what it's like to be . . . [for example] this person's shoulders are hunched; therefore, he/she must be feeling this.

Instead of learning just how to read body language, students learn how to use all of their sensory modalities and empathic capacity to imagine what clients are feeling. As they do this repeatedly over time they begin to develop the kind of skills that a practicing dance/movement therapist is expected to apply to working with clients.

Students emphasized the powerfulness of experiential activities and how these activities facilitated their ability to connect theory with practice.

> She would lead a session with a specific theme, set up an experience, and give direction for students to go into some space. Students became clients. We worked through group process by experiencing it. Jane facilitated [the] verbal process to get insight into what happened. Jane would bring up what happened based on what people would say.

Another student shared that it was the nature of her instruction that helped her apply classroom learning to clinical practice.

> Rather than expecting us to . . . memorize techniques, she trained us on how to observe and use body and feelings to connect with patients. She trained us to focus on seeing, hearing, feeling what's happening with client, not what should I do. She stressed that we would need to walk away from our books and get into reality. She trained us to feel patients right away. If you observe clients' movements, you will understand what to do, rather than dwelling on techniques alone.

Still others reported how their training personally affected them. As a result of being trained in dance/movement therapy, one student observed that she began to "recognize the meaning embedded in stiffened visceral parts and developed more choices in interactions with people." She reported

> being able to connect the emotion of life experience with the impulse to move, to stretch, to twist, to bend, to bounce body parts and to go through certain patterns, or to start letting certain patterns evolve and develop [and that she has become] open to reflecting on what that may mean.

She was able to behave in this manner, "partly as a result of being trained because you are attuned to what's being communicated from your soma to your psyche and back and forth now." She also reported that

> [I] begin to notice if I'm having a conversation with someone, I'll find a tightness in some part of my forehead. I observe my body as I am in groups or in relationships. Not all the time, but once in a while something asserts itself at the edge of my consciousness, and I let it in and notice it. It usually flags me to some sort of place in me where I'm coming from in that conversation that some other part of me that wants to observe. I've become a much more rich, complex, and interesting person to myself in this process. It's given me more choices in how I interact with people. [Now] I can run an options list on myself and sometimes I can persuade myself that it's perfectly safe to be comfortable there. And then what goes on in that room totally changes because I have that empowerment.

Students and friends have identified a number of Jane Ganet-Sigel's teaching strengths. The mostly frequently cited practices are shown below in Table 3.8.

Table 3.8 Summary of Jane Ganet-Sigel's Teaching Strengths

1. Provides experiential activities.
2. Communicates authentically with students.
3. Provides mentoring during and after graduate studies.
4. Promotes active learning.
5. Pushes students to their growing edge.
6. Places the onus for learning on students.
7. Encourages students to develop their capacity for leadership.
8. Offers students honest feedback and appraisal.

Teaching Sandra to Become a Dance/Movement Therapist

In her lengthy career at Columbia College, Ganet-Sigel had occasion to help train many individuals as dance/movement therapists. One of her most unique students was a seventy year old woman, Sandra Begain[7], a former chair of the Chicago Dance Council and a dance teacher.

---

[7]Sandra Begain is a pseudonym.

Sandra was a real challenge. She had her own ideas since she had been a dance instructor for thirty-four years. Listening did not come easy to her. Patiently, Ganet-Sigel had to teach her that the primary role of a therapist was to help her client. She explained to Sandra that her ego had to be kept out of the picture if she had any idea of becoming a successful therapist.

While someone else was talking, often Sandra was not paying attention. Either she was busy planning or could be heard saying, "Next." However, Sandra soon learned that the therapist had specific responsibilities. First, she discovered that the therapist must carefully listen to her clients. Moreover, she learned that it was crucial to permit clients' needs and feelings to guide the therapeutic process. Sandra quickly learned that it was a grave misunderstanding for a therapist to come to a group session with any expectation of implementing a lesson plan.

Ganet-Sigel offered Sandra a framework and accompanying techniques to help her guide movement processes during group sessions.

1. Develop the ability to wait and to be with a client in a non-interfering way.
   Technique: Encourage the clients to move in ways that are satisfying to them rather than following the therapist. Explain that there is no right or wrong way to move, except that group members may not hurt themselves, others, or the therapist.

2. Establish a trusting and warm relationship with clients.
   Technique: Return phone calls in a timely manner to convey a sense of trust.

3. Participate when the whole group is dancing.
   Technique: Model how to participate in a group. The act of modeling by the therapist is important to the development of a cohesive group. For example, when Jane led group members in the circle, she also interacted with each group member during the movement. As one student observed, "Jane works hard to give her budding therapists the tools, goals, and ethics to succeed. She also gives her groups cues to prevent upsetting incidents."

4. Make sure the environment is safe and pleasant.
   Technique: Make certain that there's nothing in the client's path, so that injuries can be avoided.

5. Protect the well-being of individuals and the entire group.
   Technique: To insure the safety and well-being of the client and other group members, the therapist should interfere calmly if the client was in danger of hurting himself/herself, another group member, or the therapist.

6. Avoid taking any comment of the group members personally.

7. Be very aware of relationships with the nurses, social workers, aides, and administrators.
   Technique: Be cognizant that the procedures used in hospitals are different from those used with high functioning groups. In the beginning, when working with a low functioning group, Jane advised Sandra to always use highly structured outer

directed movements during the warm-up and pay careful attention to the sensations that clients demonstrate during this period.

8. Work together with co-workers to promote healing and well-being of clients.
Technique: Acknowledge positive behavioral changes to clients. Jane told Sandra that: "Even if there is the slightest improvement, be sure to acknowledge this to the client. Be positive, yet truthful with clients." In this way, the therapist can help clients build their egos and also build a therapeutic alliance and trusting relationship.

She instructed Sandra about the process of initiating a group session and offered the following advice.

When the group is preparing to move, begin with a warm-up period. To prepare clients for a warm-up on their own, tell the group that they are now going to explore breathing and that their hands are to feel what happens to the body when they are breathing properly. Explore with the group what can be done with isolated parts: the head, the arms, the legs, the torso. When clients are more experienced and discover the kind of warm-up that their bodies need, then clients can be allowed to use their own warm-up.

Often it helps a client to close his/her eyes during warm-up or during a movement. However she cautioned Sandra that: "It is wrong to have the client close his/her eyes if unconscious material is overwhelming, frightening, or if painful memories intrude. In these instances, it is not safe for such clients to go inside." As the clients do their warm-up, Sandra was advised to observe and listen carefully and choose music that fit the mood of the group: folk music, Latino, or waltz.

Ganet-Sigel urged Sandra to enrich the clients' movement vocabulary and encourage them to let different parts of their bodies lead the movement. She suggested that:

The impulses may be the head, the shoulder, the hip. Give clients an opportunity to share what images they felt as they moved: mother with a baby; I felt like an elf; I felt like a bird; I felt like an elephant. Ask the group how it felt to share the images.

Ganet-Sigel recommended that "to help clients get more experience in witnessing others, have each member mirror one another's movement even though the movement may not always use obvious balance." After mirroring one another, Ganet-Sigel suggested that Sandra ask clients: "How did it feel to be seen or to witness what someone else was sharing?" Ganet-Sigel also advised Sandra to ask clients if their images changed and whether their movement was being observed by others or they were observing another client move. She asked Sandra to "have clients explore that difference."

Ganet-Sigel encouraged Sandra to have clients relate to one another. "Have clients go around the circle and use nonverbal action to communicate with other clients." This technique is used to help clients become more comfortable when he/she is seen or witnessing other group members move. Ganet-Sigel suggested that clients transfer an imaginary object from one person to another or move with transitional objects like a chair, scarf, wand, or fan. She also reminded Sandra that "It is not wrong to have a silence in movement or in listening." Ganet-Sigel urged Sandra to avoid countertransference, and advised that: "[If you] discover that the group is dealing with [your] material, begin to do less, intervene less, and wait longer."

To ensure that clients could offer and receive feedback from one another in an appropriate manner, Sandra was urged to monitor the feedback and ensure that they were compassionate and tactful to one another. "Transformation may occur when the client feels comfortable moving and being seen — also when he/she is witnessing others move." Ganet-Sigel recommended that: "The feedback at the closing [of a session] should be initiated by the group members." She reminded Sandra that: "Often clients are not always helped by the therapist's feedback, instead they may be helped by a group member's contribution."

Throughout her internship, Ganet-Sigel urged Sandra to listen and observe her clients thoughtfully. With patience and clear guidance, she helped Sandra become a successful therapist in her work with geriatric patients.

Conclusion

Ganet-Sigel offers a broad eclectic base in her teaching about the methodologies and techniques of doing dance/movement therapy. Her instructional process is guided by a solid conceptual model of learning that is rooted in a humanistic, constructivist approach and complemented by formative assessment techniques to promote effective learning. By giving students an opportunity to experience theories and methods and practice ideas and techniques in simulated groups, Ganet-Sigel's students learn by example.

Ganet-Sigel helps students translate classroom learning for use in the clinical setting by a variety of methods including: modeling, group discussions, critiques of simulated group work, and coaching during internship experiences. She places the onus for learning squarely upon students' shoulders but is available to help students make sense out of their learning experiences.

As a teacher, Ganet-Sigel is acknowledged as one who honors her students' interests in particular therapeutic approaches and accepts their candor. While she is known as a tough instructor, students regard her as a supportive and strong mentor. Following graduation, she welcomes former students into the profession and freely accepts them as fellow colleagues.

CHAPTER 4

The Impact of a Practicing Dance/Movement Therapist

Guiding Questions

1. What can students of dance/movement therapy learn from Ganet-Sigel's work as a therapist?

2. How has dance/movement therapy been used to help the clients described in this chapter?

3. What are some of the techniques that were instrumental in the clients' recovery?

4. In what ways did Ganet-Sigel use observation to facilitate clients' awareness?

5. What type of therapeutic environment did Ganet-Sigel offer her clients?

Motion . . . influences the body-image and leads from a change in the body-image to a change in the psychic attitude. . . . There is so close an interrelation between the muscular sequence and the psychic attitude that not only does the psychic attitude connect up with the muscular states, but also every sequence of tensions and relaxations provokes a specific attitude (Schilder, 1950, p. 208). But every emotion is either connected with expressive movement or at least with impulses towards them. Every emotion therefore changes the body image (Schilder, 1950, p. 210).

In her private practice, Ganet-Sigel has worked primarily with what she calls the "normal neurotic." Characteristically this population is comprised of individuals who are functioning in society, yet collectively they seem to have issues that interfere with their ability to utilize comfortable coping mechanisms. Examples of these issues include trust, intimacy, autonomy, role identification, separation, aggression, socialization, loneliness, sexual dysfunction, and self-esteem, among others. For the new dance/movement therapist or the student who hasn't been involved in clinical work for many years, it is natural to have many unanswered questions about what patients experience. Just as the effective educator seeks to understand and assess students' experiences so that he/she may sharpen his/her skills, the good dance/movement therapist needs to come to understand the patients' perspectives, so that he/she can be effective in guiding clients towards health. Although there is no substitute for direct hands-on experience and developing an appreciation for the clients' felt experiences, this type of expertise can be obtained over many years of work in the field. The following chapter will provide insight for students who want to understand the potential of dance/movement therapy to catalyze healing and the range of outcomes and experiences with a variety of clients. Using vignettes of clients' experiences drawn from her work over a thirty-year period, the authors provide a means to illustrate Ganet-Sigel's approach to dance/movement therapy.

In this chapter, the authors describe how the process of dance/movement has helped many private practice clients lead a more functional and healthy life. The reader will learn how clients' therapeutic interactions with Ganet-Sigel have led to deep and fundamental changes, including both a strengthened sense of self and well-being. A discussion of how specific techniques can be utilized during the process of dance/movement is also described.

Why do clients chose to enter into the process of dance/movement therapy? In interviews with current and former clients, we learned that the reasons for selecting this modality ranged from a peripheral acquaintance with Ganet-Sigel's work to unsuccessful relationships with verbal therapists. For example, one client chose to work with Ganet-Sigel at the urging of his wife, who was one of her students. He shared that: "My wife was adamant that I go to Jane. [I] consented because [this] was the lowest point of my life." He also related that:

> I wasn't a person that would have remotely ever gone to a therapist . . . in reality, things were already falling apart. . . . [However] as long as there was money there, everybody was satisfied back home here so it was a typical kind of thing where — we're able to patch over things because of money, that solved our problems. So in reality, we probably had problems . . . but . . . not in a million years would [I] have ever gone and sought out help. So the only reason I went to Jane was because my wife really insisted on it. At least to go once and see how it was.

Another client remarked that he chose to work with Ganet-Sigel because: "My wife was working with Jane, so it seemed natural. I had already [unsuccessfully] experienced art and verbal therapies." One former student who later become a client shared that: "My studies in dance/movement therapy made this a natural choice. Dance/movement therapy has a holistic view of mind and body." Another client who had also been one of her students shared that she worked with Ganet-Sigel and a verbal therapist simultaneously. Another woman sought Ganet-Sigel's help because she had experienced physical and sexual abuse and was experiencing depression. Having been in therapy since she was sixteen with at least five verbal therapists, she had worked on these issues for a long time. She recounted that she had grown weary of trying to establish a healthy therapeutic alliance with verbal therapists.

> I have not had any results. In many cases, I got worse. And in one case, in particular with the male that I was working with, I became more concerned about his well-being than I was about mine. And so I began to notice something very peculiar about verbal therapists — that I was going to . . . that in many cases they were as needing of emotional support as I was. And that disturbed me . . . because it was bleeding over into my sessions.

One former student who is now a practicing dance/movement therapist began her work in dance/movement therapy following graduation, although she believed that she had no issues which necessitated therapy. Instead she was convinced that therapy would be a learning experience. Her rationale for seeking therapy was that:

> I wanted to be a sponge and learn as much as I could from Jane. To become a dance therapist, [I believe that] one should have at least to experience it first hand. And I was going to work on my mind and body.

Another client reported that years of psychotherapy had not only lead to further dysfunction, but that she felt her body was exploding from rage. She concluded that verbal therapy was not beneficial to her and that it offered her neither solace nor an outlet for intense feelings. Threatening to commit suicide, she insisted she needed to work with a dance/movement therapist.

Another woman made an appointment because she was experiencing trouble in her marriage. She stated that ". . . I had a big fight with my husband, and I got terribly drunk, and it scared me. I knew that I needed to see someone immediately." Frightened by her unhealthy use of alcohol, she felt she needed the help of a therapist. At first she was very conflicted about a friend's recommendation that she see Ganet-Sigel.

> I know initially I thought, "God, I don't need to learn to dance." Here I'm like just totally devastated . . . [and my friend] is telling me to go to a dance person. I wasn't really sold on dance therapy, because I didn't even know what it was. This sounds kind of like a gimmick, [I thought] I think I need more than this, but I'm going to go to her and just see what happens. . . . I went with a lot of skepticism. But yet at the same time, she said that this woman really helped her. And I just — I was feeling real desperate.

What type of healing have dance/movement therapy clients experienced? One man shared that the therapeutic process "catalyzed my need for affiliation, [and to be] in a significant relationship. [The awareness I gained in therapy] catalyzed my need to establish balance in my home and family lives." From his work with Ganet-Sigel, another client reported that although he recognized that his struggle would be ongoing, he felt that he had gained the necessary tools to cope with issues. The therapeutic process was not always comfortable for him. As a result of engaging in the movement process he described that he felt:

> . . . [dance/movement therapy] forced me to something unnatural, move, [and] let my body go. [However I] let myself go and just go with my feelings, [and] not worry about being judged by others, (no rejection occurred) . . . to encounter another person (non-sexually) [and] recognize that there were no constraints. [This actually] heightened my awareness of how I respond to my children and others. [Now I am] trying to be more aware of how things affect my children and become more reflective.

He also reported learning how to "value [his] partnership with my wife, to trust myself, and others, and talk about things" as a result of his therapy.

Describing how the process helped her feel more grounded, one woman reported that dance/movement:

> . . . gave me continuous strength and balance. [Now] I am stronger, more self-assured, more assertive and less afraid to take risks. [My work with Jane] has given me impetus to conduct a more productive and healthy lifestyle and taught me to utilize better and good judgment. [Dance/movement therapy has] given me tools and knowledge of when to exercise them. [It] has enhanced my life in many aspects. Because of the work [I did] with Jane and the group, [I now] have a solid self-worth/image of myself.
> . . . Jane's capacity for empathy and intuition were magnificent. [She had an extraordinary facility for] meeting and greeting people where they are. Jane facilitates and allows individuals to experience self-discovery. [I] would not be the individual I am today without the influence of Jane and the group.

Another woman reported that she had felt totally rejected by her biological mother and lived with that pain until her late 30's when she finally began to work with Ganet-Sigel. She related the impact of working with her in a therapist-client relationship.

> Jane was a powerful woman in my life — overwhelmingly nurturing and safe. [I] felt some kind of enormous safety with her that allowed me to experience a range of feelings I had never been aware of. [She] provided [the] missing developmental experiences you wanted, needed, yearned for. [She] provided holding, [and a] nurturing environment; [more importantly, she] provided approval and validation of me.

An African-American man who felt caught between two worlds, his family of origin and corporate White America, tried to blend into the corporate world. He behaved in ways so that he would not be perceived like a "typical black," reflect negatively on black people, or in some way pass on the stereotype that he presumed that white people had about black people. Among the ways that he tried to lessen a focus on his blackness were that he came into his office very early to compensate for that fact that most people thought that black people were always late. He also made sure that he was as grammatically correct as possible, just because he didn't want people to think he was incapable of communicating. At times he found himself wondering if the reason that he married a white woman was to somehow prove that he was not a typical black person. His struggles centered in part around his perceptions of his successfulness in his personal and professional lives, and in portraying the image at least on the surface, that his life appeared to be going pretty well. Sharing how his work in dance/movement impacted him, he reported that the process:

> . . . caused me to look at issues without stereotyping [and] to be free of associating my behavior with others. [Here I] began to see myself as an individual [and] let go of feelings that I had to continuously repackage myself. [I] became less angry [and] confronted messages from childhood; I felt I was an aberration within my family of origin. [I began to] let go of feelings of wariness and being on guard for everything.
>
> I think Jane's sensitivity to what it meant to be black I think was . . . probably as significant as her technique or her skill. I think she understood — again being Jewish and being a Jewish woman, she seemed to have a particular sensitivity to what I may or must have been encountering myself. I think that sensitivity made her very credible. And so being credible for me — and we talked about that, how important credibility is for me. Most of my life has been in states of being credible myself, so when I'm talking to other people or working with other people, I'm always looking for what makes them credible in the roles that they're at that point in time in. So Jane being able to understand the plight and dynamic that I had been in conflict with . . . her understanding made her very credible. That credibility allowed me to kind of turn myself over to her and let her see me and certainly work me through certain particular motions. But I think that probably more than anything else established our relationship.

While confronting his views and preconceived notions about who he believed he was as a person, as a man, as a black man, and living in the world, he also had to confront some messages he received during childhood.

> . . . probably the most work that I was doing was the messages that my parents gave me and the environment that I grew up probably reinforced. "You know, black people aren't supposed to be successful, they aren't supposed to be achievers or they're not supposed to aspire for anything beyond whatever the typical black was supposed to have.". . . A lot of problems [ensued] for me because I wasn't sure you all knew what typical meant. And then I felt like I was kind of an aberration because I was not content

with being typical. My brothers and sisters, of which there are seven, would challenge me and ask why do I want to be different . . . [be in an] interracial marriage and live in a suburb outside of Chicago.

I guess my parents and that environmental message was "Always be careful, don't overstep, don't [let them] know that you're anything other than just a typical old black male, because if you shine out more, they're going to try to destroy you." So [I felt] . . . wary and . . . always on guard for everything, for literally everything.

Another client described how her work in dance/movement helped her feel validated. The dance movement process: "gave me integrity; a sense of what I am. [It] made my choices wider. I am not as judgmental with myself and others." Feeling affirmed through the process of working with Ganet-Sigel, one woman described how therapy impacted her.

She truly cares for us. She looks at us while we're moving. She promotes trust and nurturing. [During therapy there is a] transference of mother, and her strength. [Moreover] being in the here and now with you gave sense of acknowledgment and authentic response. [She] would speak her mind and be truthful.

How does dance/movement therapy help clients experience fundamental and deep changes in the quality of their lives? The following excerpts from client interviews reveal the significance of the dance/movement therapeutic process. One woman commented that:

I made the most challenging journey of my life [and] averted an early death. [Dance/movement therapy] . . . allowed me to have some safety in my body. . . . Now if I hadn't been able to trust the process that I began with Jane, I don't think I would be able to trust the people that are coming into my life now to help me. Because I had people available to me for many years to help me and I just couldn't stay with any kind of process because it was just too painful physically. Trust in the dance/movement therapy process facilitated trust in others. [It] allowed me to see and feel beauty in my body and movement [and] to absolve me of guilt for bodily abuse. Dance/movement therapy offered me a safe, and non-judgmental environment [and helped me] learn to see myself in another light.

Victims of physical and sexual abuse may experience a mechanism that shuts down the body and the mind, so that one doesn't have to relive or face the pain again. The pain may be so intense for clients who have weak ego structures that the potential to sever their psyche or experience a psychotic breakdown is significant. Dance/movement therapy provides a safe haven for clients to reveal deep-seated traumas. Ganet-Sigel's ability to accept clients in a nonjudgmental manner facilitates movement, provides a sense of safety, and encourages them to observe the beauty in their own movement. The creation of this environment is a catalyst in the healing process.

Also learning different ways of viewing herself, another client reported that her work in dance/movement therapy:

> . . . made me look at myself in other ways. Talking about move-
> ment during the verbal portion of the session [was very helpful in
> this regard]. [I] felt a mother, teacher, and trusting figure in Jane.
> Jane's nonjudgmental attitude, her recognition of when to push
> and when to lay back, her sensitivity to client's sense of neediness
> [were instrumental].

Another client shared that the process helped her to develop a "denser sense of self [and a] strengthening sense of self." As a result of her therapy, she reports that she is now able to "remain on an even keel." In fact, she finds that it is "difficult to disrupt my sense of cen-teredness" because [through her work with Jane she] has [developed a] "solidified a sense of stability."

For one client, dance/movement brought about a new understand-ing of his predominate conflict and the range of choices he could make concerning his own beliefs.

> I think the first part of working with Jane was coming to under-
> stand I really did bring quite a bit to my personal life as well as
> my working professional life. I tend to be a perfectionist. I tend-
> ed to not hear something positive or a compliment, thinking that
> there was an ulterior purpose to the compliment or a positive
> statement about me. I tended to just put myself down and conse-
> quently negate what others would say and as result, put others
> down. So I guess working with Jane really opened me up to, to
> my own positiveness, and helped me get past the BS I was kind of
> like building, incorporating into, into my own identity.
>
>   Also I think what happened is that Jane really forced me to
> look at some of the stereotypes that either consciously or uncon-
> sciously, willingly, unwillingly [that] I bought into about being
> black and about who I was. . . . When I say stereotypes, I'm talk-
> ing the ability to the [create] self-fulfilling prophecies, the inabil-
> ity to compete with white males and other people, the feeling that
> if I'm there, it must be because they're making a special case for
> me. All of the crap that was going on about that time, and some
> way, somehow I bought into. And part of it meant that I had to
> work harder than everybody else. Now there's a truth to that, but
> to the point that I had really incorporated it into just about every-
> thing I did. I think it had caused me to look very suspiciously at
> my own marriage. So I think that's probably the biggest help and
> support that I got out of Jane.

Suffering from intense anger and conflicts around his own identity, he related how Ganet-Sigel helped him find resolution.

> . . . repackaging myself continually to the point I wasn't even sure
> what I had repackaged myself into. I wasn't the guy in the gray

flannel suit. I wasn't the guy in the dashiki. I . . . didn't know what I was . . . it'd got to the point that what kind of clothes did I buy, and why was I buying the clothes. . . . I ended up buying them because I had to worry about what the effect was going to be, what the social impact was going to be. And, . . . it just started to make me even resent myself . . . and I just knew at that point that I couldn't go on living that way. So that's where Jane was probably, again, very helpful.

Proclaiming the catalytic aspect of dance/movement therapy, one woman shared how the therapeutic process helped her make a variety of major life decisions because she: "got in touch with gut-wrenching, crying, rageful feelings. [Jane] provided [the] kind of nurturance and mothering that I needed." Working in dance/movement, as she described gave:

me some internal feelings of some power; of having rights; of having and voicing my own thoughts. I stood up to my husband [and began to] separate my feelings from past reactions to similar behavior by my mother. [Also I] became in touch with what [had been] modeled for me by my parents and what I was reliving in my marriage. I went back to school and got my Ph.D. in clinical psychology, encouraged my son to become more autonomous [and I learned to] trust my gut.

The process of dance/movement helped her make "a tremendous connection with my head and my body that I never had. My body was just like totally foreign to me. . . . I just couldn't move it . . . and so the body freedom really came along very much with the feeling of power and feeling of choices and feeling that I had a right to please myself, and the freedom with my body came gradually at that same time." Working with Ganet-Sigel helped her get in touch with herself and fortified the belief that she had some power and an entitlement of rights.

. . . I don't think I felt like I had any rights. My husband had all the rights. My parents had all the rights. . . . I didn't feel like I had any right to anything of my own. Even my own thoughts. . . . I was kind of successful professionally, but still . . . I didn't feel like I still had any power. I couldn't tell my husband, "No, don't hang that picture there, hang it over here." My husband knew best. I felt like he knew best about everything. And he was . . . kind of authoritarian. And so we worked well together [because] I didn't fight back. I still have lots kind of guilt feelings that I didn't go for some help sooner. My son was two, my daughter was four. I feel like those first four years of my marriage and my children's lives were pretty bad. I don't know. Maybe not so bad, but I mean, I didn't have any right to stand up for myself. I didn't have any right to stand up for my kids. My husband was pretty verbally abusive to our kids when they were tiny. I was too scared to stand up to him. And now, I . . . would have a gut-sick reaction when he would be angry, just like I would with my mother. But then . . . all that changed. I was able to stand up to him. I didn't have gut reactions any more when he would be angry. I could like separate myself from it, and tell him to go to hell, and leave, and do whatever I had to do. And then it sent him in to see Jane.

During the process of dance/movement therapy, she became in touch with what was modeled by her family of origin and what she was currently reliving in her own marriage. As she began to move and get in touch with her viscera and experience feelings, the rage compacted into her body and began to erupt. Freed from this imprisonment, she gradually began to speak her mind and make choices that were more self-satisfying.

> My experience with Jane was that she was just huge. That she was six feet tall. She was overwhelmingly nurturing and supportive and safe. . . . I think I just felt some kind of enormous safety with her that allowed me to just experience a range of feelings that I had never even been aware of at all . . . she just was a very, very, very significant person in my life. And she just always seemed to be able to move in and help me in a way that just was [what I needed]. . . .

Exhibiting a remarkable capacity to be empathic and to provide clients with the missing developmental things they wanted and needed and yearned for so badly in childhood, Ganet-Sigel offered them as a matter of course.

> She gave me the kind of holding, nurturing environment that I had never experienced in my life . . . and approval. . . . I don't think I ever had approval . . . one of the biggest things that I worked out in the rage against my mother. I don't ever, ever remember of having one iota of approval from my own mother. Until maybe she was eighty and I was fifty or something. But there was the longing for approval. I think [this] was really a big thing in my relationship with Jane . . . I just felt her approval of me and validation of me, and I don't believe I had ever had it in my life before.

Able to change his view of himself, another client reported that he no longer felt judged and filtered [by others] through racial and cultural lenses. He related that he: "no longer carried [the issue of] race on my shoulders and overcompensated. [I] relinquished feelings that my own behavior might reflect negatively on black people as a whole."

Because of her experiences as a dance/movement therapy client, another woman commented that she had:

> become flexible [enough] to tolerate stress in my active life [and] able to sit quietly without sinking into fugue. I am more forgiving of myself. [Dance/movement therapy] gave me tools to engage in process of reworking the way I view myself.

Sharing how she believed that her therapeutic work affected the dynamics of her family relationships, one client revealed that: "[I] experienced changes in relationship with family. [Now I] feel whole and stable [as well as] emotionally and psychologically grounded. [I] learned to be good to myself [and to focus on] changing myself rather than others."

One client related that the therapeutic process helped him find other parts of himself, that he no longer felt invincible, and that he experienced a complete change of attitude. After having dealt with a sense of remorse for unethical conduct that resulted in losing his job, he reported that he now has a better relationship with his wife and family, and sees himself as a good person in an ethical framework. "[I became] more peaceful [and] realized that the end results don't supersede the means. Money isn't the only thing that matters."

Another client reported the range of healing she experienced as a dance/movement therapy client.

> [I was] in therapy with Jane for over ten years. [Now I] feel healthy and strong, not needing to please others, [I am] able to balance others' needs without undermining [my] own [instead of] needing to be the "good little girl". [I have experienced] improved relations with family and others; [my] self-confidence and judgment has improved. [I have a] refined and solidified sense of centeredness and stability and direction. [I am] healthier, [having] moved from stagnation to positive action.

The therapeutic process, although uncomfortable at times, helped one client work through issues and confront stereotyped views that he had been raised with and accepted without question.

> Dance/movement therapy versus actually sitting down with other forms of therapists or psychiatrists or whatever broke down a lot of barriers. And when I was entered in to the group, [instead of] just working with Jane . . . and [had] to physically . . . touch people and move with people . . . my issues with women and/or dealing with a man [in] that way was just very foreign to me. . . . I think I was raised in a fairly shielded type of home . . . with three brothers and obviously my parents. But my mother was not one to — not like you don't disrespect women but it . . . she's a person that believed that, a man works, a woman stays at home . . . what's the word? Not conservative, but just an old-fashioned type . . . [this was the] way we were raised. So I never had a woman who was a friend. Either it was a girlfriend, or I had my men friends.
>
> It was a long process . . . at first it was just breaking down my barriers and my old-time beliefs, of just allowing me to do that and opening my mind up to . . . just believe in it and let it happen. And it took a long time, but all of a sudden, I think half way through it, things started clicking that this the movement and the closeness, trusting other people, whether it be a man or a woman, trusting someone that I might not necessarily have a ten-year-old

relationship with, but you get to know someone very well in that kind of atmosphere even though it's — most of it's nonverbal.

By confronting some of the myths and beliefs he held, he became touched by the humanism of what other people were going through as well as their compassion and empathy towards him. He reported that he confronted his sexual feelings towards women and his inability to develop platonic friendships with women. Commenting about the important role that Ganet-Sigel played in this process, he shared that:

> . . . I felt a mother figure [in Jane], a combination of a teacher, a mother figure, just a lot of different things. If I didn't have the trust in her, I would not have been able to come around like I did, [if it were not for the role that Jane played] . . . a mother figure that was not judging me.

Through his therapy, he explored the preconceived notions he had about the appropriateness of physicality towards men and women and how to behave in the company of people he found unattractive or otherwise might not care to even talk with. Much of his therapy focused on helping him consider the impact of how he was raised and how his beliefs affected what he felt were appropriate roles for men and women.

One client who felt absolutely certain that she had no problems soon learned that although she came to therapy for the wrong reasons, it was a good decision.

> When I first came into therapy, I thought I was healthy. And then as the process went on, I started to realize there are parts of me that can change. I realized how I was unsatisfied in some things and working with Jane, I was able to move from being stagnant to actually putting into motion this change and feeling the wellness from within. Jane facilitated that process.

Describing the connection between movement and cognition, this client stated that:

> The "dynamic process" of hearing and sharing with other people's experiences [was pivotal in my emerging awareness]. . . . Jane would have us experience similar and different suggestions and learn viscerally our patterns and learn how we could alter our unhealthy patterns.

Over time, her experience with new patterns of movement lead to a visceral sense of comfort. Doing these patterns and different kinds of movement within the security, community, and love of the group gave her the confidence and the awareness and the insight to say, "Hey this really is okay."

> I remember the effect of the movement and Jane's comments afterwards. The group, under Jane's guidance, had some mem-

bers become agitators, and she had us exaggerate the movement. I got such a thrill from just playing this different role and the movement and being able to just stick my tongue out at other members of the group. I was really getting on their nerves. Jane facilitated the process of making connections of mind and body by her comments of her observations during the discussion part of group. She saw a change in my body attitude and the excitement in my face. It was like an affirmation of a part of me that I wasn't used to or should I say never had an opportunity to feel the role. And it made me open my eyes. I had to confirm that excitement. Jane allowed me to experience this role without judgment, and I was able to accept this element as a part of me and to use when needed.

I could try out new roles without guilt, feel playful with it, become the role. During these transformations Jane was also able to viscerally feel my change. To hear her observations acknowledging how I moved [helped] focus [my own] realizations. . . .

At times Ganet-Sigel would suggest that clients move to words such as *push*, *pull*, *slash*, or *hit*. How did the use of words affect movement? One client described how words were used and how the process of dance/movement therapy catalyzed healing.

She'd let you be with it for awhile and not change the "word" until the sense of it is tried out. Sometimes we have to be in something that's maybe a little uncomfortable before we can understand it.

[If it weren't for my experience in dance/movement therapy] I would have never left home. I would have stayed in an awful relationship. It's just incredible how therapy opened my eyes. My relationship with my mother, it is like night and day now compared to before I was in therapy. I truly feel whole and definitely stable.

I believe [that through] the movements and discussions with Jane I learned to be good to myself, to give to myself. Movement was definitely used in "giving to self." To give and receive in this process. I realized I deserved better. For example, in the relationship or no relationship, I can give to myself and exist with myself happily, that's what helped me there. The change with my family developed out of the discussions with Jane. I learned that I can't change our family. They are going to be what they are. The only person I can change is myself. And then when my family saw the changes in me, they may not have realized it, gradually they changed in the sense of how they would interact with me, because I wasn't affected by their ways or old patterns.

Clients also reported specific aspects of their therapeutic work with Jane that promoted healing. A client who had suffered from physical abuse, sexual molestation, and battery reported that she experienced physiological changes. She claimed that the dance/movement process offered her "safety of embodiment [that facilitated the] reconnection with parts of body and psyche." Another client stated that: "[In my work with Jane I] engaged in the dance of life. [I] can't separate the way I move, feel, touch, taste, and see. [Now I] understand and can articulate these interactions and what I feel."

What techniques of dance/movement therapy were helpful to clients? One client reported how words and the suggestion of imagery helped him. "At times Jane would place written words on the board (*push, pull*). The use of the written word was a nonthreatening way to move into emotion on a motoric level. Also she use offered images that facilitated movement."

Observing movement patterns was facilitative for another client. Ganet-Sigel's observations of this client's movements led him to look at parts of his life. He realized that he was holding in, protecting self, regulating, controlling, and shutting off feelings. As a result of what this client learned about his movement, he began to understand that he brought a lot of stereotyped messages to his personal and professional life.

> [The] movement allowed me not to always have to search for words. After individual therapy, I went to group therapy and felt their acceptance of me, a willingness to help me, validation of me as a person, not as a black male or overcompensator [and the] love of a larger community and a mixture of people who accepted me as a person. [The therapeutic process] opened me up to my own positiveness [and] forced me to look at some stereotypes. [I] confronted messages and feelings about being black in a white corporation and in a biracial marriage.
>
> The movement — allowed me just to not have to search for words all the time. And that probably may have been the biggest change for me. I think after a little bit, she began this look [and] as she saw things that I was doing, she said, "Okay, what is this all about?" . . . "You seem like this, you're. . . . "
>
> I remember this one statement she made about my pelvis being so rigid. And I said, "You know, I think part of that has to do with everyone always used to say black people were great dancers and all that. And I guess I'm trying to show them that I wasn't. By showing that I wasn't a great dancer, I was not black. So we just talked about how [I went] around overcompensating. And we just saw how that one part of movement really kind of fit into a whole lot of other areas of my life.
>
> Really, that whole issue about overcompensating and even overcompensating to the point that I would even stop other parts of my body in order to not let anyone put me into this stereotype. So I think as one example, that's probably one way in which her observations of my movement got me to look at what I was doing in other parts of my life. And I think also just being able to take that very concrete part of my objectively observable part of me and say, "Here's what you did again," and processing those things that I was doing, that I knew that I didn't know that I was doing, but certainly I could recall them after she brought them to my attention, began to look at them from the standpoint of how I was holding things in and trying to protect myself and defend myself . . .

Another client reported that the act of working viscerally and kinesthetically, using the tools of the body instead of just talking from the neck up, "developed my confidence, gave me courage, and made me assertive." Explaining the powerfulness of the therapeutic process, one client revealed that:

> [It] gave me a feeling of power. [I] engaged in exorcism [and] made connections between my head and my body. Body freedom accompanied feelings of power and choices and that I had a right to please myself. [I was] able to internalize a lot of Jane in me. [I] could hear her voice in me. [The therapeutic process with Jane provided me with] consistency, always there, always safe.

When asked to describe how the process of dance/movement therapy promoted a sense of well-being, many of the clients' responses related to the type of person Ganet-Sigel is and the kind of therapeutic environment that she provided. One client observed that "Jane fosters change. Jane emphasizes and models balance, establishing a sense of community. She celebrates and encourages engagement in a variety of life experiences."

> Jane has a strong character. She lends a strong, supportive ego; she has a commitment to accentuating the positive and the present. She provides a holding environment. She meets clients on the plane in which they reside. She has empathy, yet challenges clients.
>
> She was in it with me. Right on my level, helping me through. Someone who was truly a good person, who was there to help me. Could trust her implicitly. She instilled trust and confidence in me. I would recommend dance/movement to others. She helped [me] make therapeutic decisions on my own. [I] felt in control of therapeutic process.

Others described how she helped them change their sense of self by opening up their minds to different ways of being and living and different qualities of life experiences.

> I think the strongest way was that — was through her own strong nature and character. Because one of the things that happens in therapy, in the therapeutic process, is that the client or the patient more or less "borrows" the ego of the therapist. That's actually how the process works. It's sort of, like I said, putting someone in intensive care and putting a Band-Aid on or a cast on somebody until they can heal. And Jane's character is very, very strong. And I think because of that it really lends itself to people like me who were so self-hating and self — negative towards the self — that, you know, I don't know that I even could have fathomed any positive self within myself. And for Jane — she always relates to the positive. She is not against people examining their past, but she seems to be more committed to people flourishing in the present and in the future. And, as I said, I think it's her strong personal character that really lends itself to some very shattered egos.

Ganet-Sigel provides a holding environment for clients as well as a place to be nurtured, but she doesn't thrust things upon clients. Instead she meets and greets clients on the plane on which they reside. In and of itself, this style creates an inherent sense of comfort for clients who work with her and the realization that she is receptive to their needs. She doesn't attempt to reinterpret clients' felt sense of reality. She carefully observes clients and attunes herself to the messages that they communicate viscerally. In fact, that was one of the purposes for which dance/movement therapy was invented. One client suggested Ganet-Sigel's training with Marian Chace and being part of the invention of dance/movement therapy qualified her as a "master dance/movement therapist" which was an important qualification in her decision to work with her.

> I think that there are certain people in life that by virtue of their own character and their own personality and their training — more or less being in the right place at the right time — conveys upon them my title of "Master." And in Jane's case, it was very important for me to work with Jane because I entered the whole odyssey of self-awareness in my mid-years. I've always felt since then that if I'm going to work I need to work with whoever is what I consider a master in a field or a teacher because I don't have the luxury of time that I had in my twenties to wade through the hierarchy, so to speak. I don't want that to sound arrogant, but it really was a matter of survival at that point.

Describing Ganet-Sigel's honesty as an asset, another client stated that:

> I think with Jane there's actually another piece to her, too, that makes her very unique and that is that she doesn't mince words or actions. I think that often in therapy what happens with some therapists is that they become so conditioned to compassion and empathy that they actually become what I would call "a little wimpy."

Her facility in knowing how to respond to the individuality of each client was observed by another client.

> When I worked with Jane in group therapy, I thought it was remarkable how she could figure it out and the sensitivity she exhibited towards peoples' needs and their inherent needs for certain qualities of communication. She seemed to become immediately attuned to people's vulnerability. As a result she would respond in ways that wouldn't cause a person with a weak structure to break down.

Concurring with this point of view, another client explained that:

> I think it is because Jane has this capacity for empathy and because she's just sort of magnificently intuitive in such a powerful way that helps you to feel acknowledged and recognized, you feel a trust. And that you can let your guard down and talk with

her and tell you things that you couldn't tell another living soul or would fear to tell another living soul.

One woman commented that she felt that Ganet-Sigel really cared for her clients and demonstrated that sense of caring in an actionable manner.

> The movement is her way of saying I care enough about you to take the time to look at you, to hear you and not let you hide behind your words, to confront your movement, to tell you how your movement is in conflict with what you say and what you say you believe in. Here's a change in your behavior, a change I feel you need to see and talk about — that must be significant.

Concurring with this viewpoint, another client observed that:

> I truly feel she cares for us in group. It's not a false care. I feel that she really listens. She really looks at us when we're moving, and she sees the dynamic of it. She is truly present. When we sit down to process, I could sense that she is open. . . . There isn't a hidden agenda. I feel that she promotes a feeling of trust that allows myself to open up more. And I feel loved. It's this true sense of caring and therapeutic nurturing. And also being strong. There was a transference of "Mother," but she is more of the healing figure and guide. So she played several roles that helped me which makes her a superb therapist for having all these qualities.
>
> She would speak her mind. I don't feel like she holds back. She's going to be very truthful of what she's observing. It's like you needed to hear certain things. So definitely she was in the "here and now," and I think that's the only way it would work. If you don't have that, connections will not happen.

Another client shared how her work led to positive behavioral changes.

> [Dance/movement therapy] obliterated self-destructive behavior and replaced it with positive things. [There is a] wonderful underpinning with dance/movement therapy. [I could] not really talk myself through things.

One client described her work ethic as a therapist. "Jane Ganet-Sigel is a taskmaster. She does not allow anyone, I think, who really is willing to come and work with her completely not to change." However she aptly suggested that the process of change also

> depends on how willing the person is to work on themselves, because she isn't about telling people what to do. But the thing that I think is her greatest gift is her — what I'll call "normalcy." . . . She is very committed to people having a balanced life. She's very committed to her own family and to family commitments and a sense of community and sharing. She's not a "lone ranger" therapist. She's not interested, I don't think, in people becoming this self-evolved, self-absorbed human being. Actually, I found after

working with her that I had more of a hunger to have what I would have called previously a quote "normal life." A spouse and, you know, relationships with my family and all the kind of things that seem normal to people who are untroubled but [to] most of us who have been troubled seem almost unattainable.

Sometimes the body has been deadened and visceral responses get repressed. Dance/movement therapy reawakens the body, the senses, the emotions, fear and anger, repression, and the energy used to repress emotion. The therapeutic process helps clients learn to separate their childhood fears and felt reality as an adult and lends itself to a lessening of the intensity of visceral reactions. One client described the therapeutic process as an opportunity to get in touch with one's own viscera. "Going back into the body, one develops awareness, mindfulness, things get cleared away, the clearing becomes more thorough." Another client shared that therapy helped him:

break down barriers, especially related to [my] perceptions of women. [I] confronted issues of touch and movement with other men and women and relinquished old beliefs. [I] began to trust others [and was] able to let myself go. [I] experienced warmth and compassion. [I also] confronted [my] feelings of love and affections [for other woman in the group] but realized action wasn't necessary.

Describing Ganet-Sigel's ability to facilitate healing, another client shared that: "She is nurturing, knowledgeable, [and] can facilitate others' growth. She creates a cohesive community in the group and provides a safe environment. She facilitates different members of the group so that they can facilitate others." Recalling the safe haven that Jane provided for her clients, one individual remarked that: "She became a good mother to me. I was mothered and re-mothered in the transference relationship with her. She provided a holding environment, my only safe place."

Another client shared how the movement helped her feel more integrated.

Over time, movement illuminated connections of how body can move and make me feel more confident. Doing simulations in group therapy produced "interactions with family members." Through different suggestions, subconsciously or somatic unconsciously, I started to realize (through these experiences) how it felt in the body and the connection with my mind, what the experiences meant to me. Through the dynamic process of hearing, sharing, I learned viscerally about my patterns and how to alter unhealthy patterns. Movement patterns over time created a visceral sense of comfort. Movement group discussions with Jane helped me make connections of what I felt and meant. Her observations about change in body movements were affirming, allowing me to explore a role without judgment. I could try on roles without guilt. Hearing her observations were acknowledgments of realizations.

Vignettes

The following vignettes describe the experiences that Michelle and Racquel had during their therapy with Ganet-Sigel. Michelle, a Caucasian and a former nun, married an African-American. She reported that she felt rejected by her biological mother and vacillated between feelings of intense anger and sadness as she constantly sought her mother's approval. During her therapy, she went back to school and earned her doctorate in clinical psychology. Today she is a practicing psychotherapist.

The Case of Michelle

I had been in a convent for many years, and I remember one second of therapy that I would like to share with you. It stands out in my mind, one moment that I can just remember. You know, that at the beginning of therapy, there's a lot of direction by Jane, and working out feelings. I remember I was laying — I was lying on the floor. My mother would correct me. This is funny, because I spent about six years with Jane working out my [feelings about my] mother. I just said "laying" and "lying." My mother would correct me right now, saying which is correct. I was laying on the floor or lying on the floor. Ask my mother, she'd tell you which one is correct. My mother always told me what was correct.

... I was waiting for her to tell me what to do, how to move. And she said, "Do what you want. Just do as you want." And I had this overwhelming awareness that I just had no idea and that even the thought of doing something, laying on that floor and doing something that was what I wanted to do was so totally foreign to me that I just started sobbing.

[I] never forgot that moment. It was just like . . . there're a lot of moments, I'm sure, but that one moment I just remember. And I think that all of sudden some kind of beginning awareness that I had some power was probably the — and I had a — another kind of funny story was, I had this one piece of music all the time, and I'd always ask for this same piece of music. And I didn't pay attention to what it was, I just knew there was something about it that I — and so finally one day, I don't know how long I used that music. And I was working on — I had tremendous, tremendous rage at my mother. I mean, absolutely just tremendous anger at my mother, who was a very cold, distant, judgmental, critical woman. And that I felt never liked me. And I went to the convent to try and please her and then still my sister then had kids, and my sister pleased her more than me, because she loved my — You know, I just never quite made it in getting my mother's approval until maybe later in my — but never then. So, . . . I would always ask for the same piece of music. And then one day, I just said, you know, I think I want to change music. I think I want something different. After that session, she said, "Do you know what that piece of music was that you were using all that time?" And I said, No, I don't know what it was. And she said, it was the theme from *The Exorcist*.

I went into group therapy with her later. . . . And so I had years of individual and then [for] quite a while, [I was] in a group. One of the things I did at the end . . . in the movement of the group. This is a little tangent, but I remember shutting everybody, physically shoving all the other group members into a closet or a little room and shutting the door and locking them in and having Jane all to myself. Which was really kind of like a powerful thing that I was able to act out, you know. She's mine I thought to myself. And it was so meaningful, because I never could displease anybody . . . and I just like physically shoved everybody.

One time we had a marathon weekend, which I very much remember in the group, and we were able to each of us have a day, just in the group, there were like six of us. And I remember my day. And I imagined that I really never dealt with my convent years, and I thought I needed to deal with leaving the convent, but I realized . . . so we got into the group and I could set up — the day was mine. I could make people who I wanted them to be and, you know . . . Oh, it was just a really, really powerful day. I realized that more than finding out "leaving the convent" was finding out "going to the convent." I had a little brother — one of the group members I made my little brother. Well, . . . I don't want to go into details except that I left home that day. I never even dealt with leaving home at nineteen and dying to my family. I mean, that's what you were supposed to do in those days, you know? And I just sobbed and sobbed and sobbed. And that wasn't my stuff with getting out of the convent, it was way back to the stuff that I had no idea was still there about even leaving home and going to the convent. And I acted this out in the group, and it was really, really powerful. That was a very powerful day. And Jane made those days safe. . . . she somehow could create an environment where a group could do that, as well as just do it with you individually. She's a very powerful woman.

Michelle recalled some of the difficult times she felt in her marriage and described how Ganet-Sigel helped both her and her family work through one particular crisis.

. . . we had a huge, huge crisis. My husband would, at times, go into rages. And I was working. My daughter called me, and I, you know, left my work, went home. He was packing his suitcase. He had physically — not exactly hurt her, but she thought he was going to. And so I put them all in the car, my son and my daughter, and I said, "We're going to see —" I called — He was in therapy with Jane at the time, and I think he had gotten . . . sometimes people get into really raw places in their therapy where all kinds of old demons are there, and I think that's what was happening to him. But anyway — didn't matter. We were all in a crisis. So I think I modeled for my kids that night.

I put them in the car and I said, "We need help. We're going to see Jane." So we drove up to see Jane, and we were there with Jane, myself and my two kids. And then he came in — because, I don't know, he got — he didn't know we were going to be there, but anyway, he came in. And he just went into a wild, wild rage right there, but it was safe. Jane knew how to handle him. She calmed him down. He and my son drove home together in the same car. You know, it was just — it was a very dramatic night. And she has a tremendous ability . . . if anybody was listening to him at that time, you'd think you should lock him up. She had the ability to contain even his rage and be there in a way for him in front of us where he calmed down and was able to, you know, as I said, ride home with my son. And it was a tremendous family event I think that — I'm sure had an impact on my kids at the time.

My children learned that we don't have to keep this in our house and pretend like it's not happening. We can go outside and get help. And I think, you know, that's the one thing, with all the mess in our family, I modeled that. That we don't have to pretend this isn't happening. We can let other people know, and we can get help.

Racquel, an African-American, entered into therapy with Ganet-Sigel when she became overwhelmed with feelings of depression. A single mother of two children, Racquel reported that she suffered from many negative messages she received as a child. As a result of her upbringing, she developed maladaptive coping mechanisms that began to impinge on leading a healthy adult life. After more than a decade in therapy with Jane, Racquel is a practicing clinical therapist.

The Case of Racquel

I perceived myself as unworthy, unpleasant, unlikable, ugly, just . . . my thing was to show deference to everyone else because I just was not good enough. And that was the message I got from home. And since then . . . I was giddy and silly, but I wasn't really assertive. I was what she called a clown. And that clown hid every imaginable difficulty and sloth that I had put upon myself. And so what she wanted to facilitate with what I wanted to facilitate and what I wanted to give birth to in myself . . . was to view myself as a worthwhile human being who was out of pain and out of fear. I was very fearful, and I was very passive. Or I was very volatile.

And we worked from there. I mean, we worked and found out where all this behavior, this maladaptive behavior came from. And we began to understand, and I began to understand, more importantly, that I didn't need it any more to survive and that I [had] needed [these behaviors] at the time I developed because that was the only way I could have survived emotionally. But that I could begin with her in that nurturing environment to actually sit down and look at myself in a different way and test very gingerly [new coping mechanisms]. It took years for me to test sometimes different ways of being. She patiently walked me through that, nurtured me through that. And the groups that I was in, we went on an adventure of self-discovery that was just extraordinary.

> . . . as a child, I don't know that I had a sense of rapprochement
> or detaching from my mother because I don't know that I was ever
> attached to her. So I didn't have any grounding. And so with Jane,
> I knew that once a week I could take myself and all my baggage
> there, and I could just be who I was. And no matter what I was
> experiencing at the time, it would be welcomed; it would be
> explored, and it would be seen through for what it was if I was ready
> to have that happen. I also knew that dancing, I knew dance from
> three years on, that dancing was my only survival. And my dances
> early on were so intense and so frenetic that I would come out
> sometimes just feeling total release . . . from just having expended
> that much energy with that much emotion attached to it. So that
> was like having a safe place to go to once a week. And I also knew
> that if I needed to call, any time day or night, that I had somebody
> then to call. Now I never really wanted to use that because I want-
> ed to respect her life, because I knew she was so busy. But I knew
> that it was there if I needed it. So I really appreciated that, too. So
> that was what I felt in terms of well-being. I felt that there was a safe
> harbor. She actually became a surrogate mom to me.

During therapy, Ganet-Sigel provided a healthy symbiosis for Racquel. However, she related that at the time she didn't experience this re-
bonding as positive.

> I think that it was healthy. At the time, I didn't recognize it as
> healthy because we were so volatile, and we had so many argu-
> ments, and . . . so I didn't perceive it as healthy, but. . . . Because
> I was so rebellious what she said and saw of me sometimes was not
> what I agreed to being. But I very slowly began to understand that
> there were some very intricate things that were happening that I
> needed to really kind of take stock of. So . . . I think that . . . she
> provided the "good enough mother,". . . she provided something
> for me to attach to. She lended ego and superego when I needed
> it. She lent me those parts of herself that in myself were unhealthy
> so that I could survive until I could replace it with something else.

During her therapeutic work, Racquel began to relive the experiences that led to the development of maladaptive coping skills and she
learned new ways to respond. Recognizing their humanity and mortality, she also learned to forgive her parents.

> There's a fundamental change that has to happen in all of us, and
> I believe it has to do with remembering. Remembering from
> whence we come. We are spiritual and soulful beings. And we step
> out into a stressful, fast-paced, very unforgiving, relentless society
> here. And very often the people who are our significant — our
> parents or our primary caregivers or our significant others are also
> embroiled in trying to survive in this. And so they don't have time
> to nurture — to give us what we need, to give us boundaries and
> limits and all that other stuff that is a very interesting dance that
> the human being has to do. And it's not instinctual.

So the fundamental thing that happened for me, the fundamental change that happened to me for Jane, with Jane, was that I
began to remember that first of all, God don't create junk. And
God created me. And that I was given a plethora of tools with
which to negotiate this bullshit out here. And that I didn't have to
buy into anything that somebody else wrote for me. And my
mother and my grandmother and my grandfather and my father
had written a script for me that no longer fit because it made me
into a sick person, my trying to fit into it. And so what I did was
I began to remember some very intrinsic truths and that is that I
have a nature that I need to call on, that I need to bring out to help
me to learn how to live in this world and to deal with the lessons
that I need to get here. [She gave me] the nets and the fishing poles
to catch the darn things and [taught] me how to put the worm on
the hook. So she gave me the tools to do this for myself, too.

Conclusion

Many clients described Ganet-Sigel as a tenacious and insightful professional who touched their lives by her unique style. Ganet-Sigel's way
of relating with clients stands as a model for the new practitioner of
dance/movement therapy. One client remarked she has the uncanny
ability to maintain the details of all her clients' histories down to notic-
ing a haircut. With a charisma and an ability to empathize, Ganet-Sigel
can step into the space with clients and let them know that she is there,
while still giving them the room necessary to experience and express
themselves. Some of the underlying themes of Ganet-Sigel's work with
clients, behaviors that are characteristic of the effective therapist, are her
capacity to: (1) form a healthy therapeutic alliance that encourages
healing, (2) engender patients' trust, and (3) offer an opportunity to
reveal, reconstruct, and reintegrate the primary relationship with their
mother figures. Many clients shared that she has a capacity for confrontation and speaking plainly. One client shared that: ". . . I think
that she's a wonderful woman, and I'm in many ways blessed and for-
tunate to have her be there at the time . . . that I was in the greatest
need." These qualities: concern for the whole client, empathy, authenticity, and relatedness are examples of the behaviors that effective
dance/movement therapists exhibit.

Through the process of dance/movement therapy, clients experience a release of repressed feelings, reveal unconscious memories and
traumas that lead to dysfunctional behavior and maladaptive coping
mechanisms, and reconstruct healthy behaviors. The movement
process brings about flowering and serves as catalysis to metamorphosis. Because movement is a nonverbal process, it helps shut off the dialogue in the head and brings about a shedding of various layers of
defense mechanisms. However it is equally important to have the client
develop a cognitive awareness so that their somatic, behavioral, and
emotional changes may be integrated into the mind, body, and spirit.

PART II

*C*ases in *D*ance/ *M*ovement *T*herapy

Introduction

Using actual case studies drawn from her clinical practice, Ganet-Sigel's therapeutic approach towards the treatment of clients in private practice is illustrated. The case studies offer fascinating insight into this mode of therapy and provide a framework for a curriculum to train dance therapists. The cases described span the duration of Ganet-Sigel's career. Each case includes a description and related analysis of the therapeutic interventions (in boldface) that were used in the therapy sessions. Chapter 5 represents a segment of her work with an autistic child at a therapeutic nursery school at the inception of her career. In Chapter 6, an overview of her therapeutic work with a young woman who suffered primarily from a borderline personality disorder but who had also been diagnosed by various therapists as schizoprehenic and manic-depressive is presented. In Chapter 7 her work with an adolescent female suffering from anorexia nervosa is described.

CHAPTER 5

Rebirthing: The Little Girl Who Thought She Was an Animal

Guiding Questions

1. *What was Leah's presenting problem?*

2. *What techniques did Ganet-Sigel use during Leah's therapy sessions?*

3 *In what ways did Ganet-Sigel apply Chace's framework for establishing therapeutic goals?*

4. *How did Leah's expression during movement and her capacity to communicate change?*

5. *In what ways did Ganet-Sigel's experience with Leah influence her work as therapist?*

His meaningful, though bizarre movements, become understandable and acceptable to others as people related themselves to him on the basis of the emotions expressed through dance action. As his feelings of isolation and his fear of lack of understanding are reduced, he is able to put aside autistic expression to an increasing degree, and this in turn seems to enable him to enter a group and function within it in a manner that is satisfying to both the patient himself, and to others in the group (Chace, 1953, p. 225).

Perhaps one of the best ways to learn about Jane Ganet-Sigel's work and dance/movement therapy is to the read the following story about a remarkable event. Early in her career, Ganet-Sigel worked at the Reed Mental Health Center in Chicago. One of her first clinical experiences was with a 4 1/2 year old girl named Leah[8] who at the time of her sessions did not speak. Her parents were divorced and for unknown reasons, Leah lived with her grandparents who were very rigid, structured, and controlling. She came to the nursery school, an outpatient setting for dysfunctional children aged 3–6. Like all children who entered the nursery school, she was placed in a classroom with two therapists and assigned to a primary therapist. The children also went to outside activities such as dance/movement therapy. Leah came to individualized dance/movement because she was not functioning well in a group.

---

[8]Names have been changed to maintain confidentiality.

One of the most striking things about Leah was that she had a very intense feeling of not being a little girl. She felt as though she were an animal. This characterization was evident not only from what she said, but from the way she carried herself. She said she was a dog and when she stood up straight, her posture and viscera revealed the striking similarity of a dog. Like a dog standing on its hind legs, her knees were slightly bent, her arms were cracked at the elbow, her wrists were cracked, her hands were rounded like a paw, and her head extended from her protruding neck.

When she came into the room for sessions, she would squat down in the corner as though she were a little puppy sitting on its hind legs, hands in front of her and head extended. Ganet-Sigel would sit the same way as Leah, but far enough away so as not to intrude on her space and or frighten her but to let her know that she was accepted. (*Accepting the client for who they are and liking them is an important therapeutic goal.*) As is characteristic of the start of each therapeutic session, Ganet-Sigel put on some music. (*Music is often used to give some timing to the session. It provides structure for people, especially the dysfunctioning client, because it offers a way of knowing the beginning and end of the session.*) As the music played, Ganet-Sigel sat next to Leah and mirrored any movements she made. Every once in a while, Ganet-Sigel changed the movement to one of her own, and would allow her wrist to release itself. Intermittently she waved to Leah like a human, rather than a dog who would move its paw.

In the beginning Leah would not accept this. Little by little as the weeks progressed, Leah began to accept her therapist. She would either wave back to Ganet-Sigel or crawl up and away from her. During this time, Leah's behavior continued to mimic that of a puppy. She would sniff Ganet-Sigel, and then move away to see if she was safe. Gradually, she crawled around the room. Ganet-Sigel mirrored this behavior as she crawled around the room with Leah. Eventually Ganet-Sigel and Leah began to play some primary baby games, like one would play with an infant, such as rubbing noses. Gradually Leah allowed Ganet-Sigel to come closer. When Leah sat up on her haunches, they played "patty cake." Subsequently Leah reached a point where she would push Ganet-Sigel over to a kneeling position and climb on top of her back to play horsie. (*Carefully and slowly the therapist established a therapeutic bond and basic trust.*)

All the while, any kind of voice Leah projected was a glatto sound. The timbre of her voice was like a growling dog. Up to this point, Leah never demonstrated a clear pure human voice. However, Leah had a way of letting Ganet-Sigel know what she wanted to do and what she didn't want to do. In fact, one time Ganet-Sigel started to play in a way that Leah did not like. Experiencing an excessive intrusion into her space, Leah went to the corner and pretended to take a hammer and nail. Leah stopped Ganet-Sigel and pretended to hammer nails into her feet. (*Symbolically, she was telling Ganet-Sigel, don't come after me, don't move, stand right here.*) Her symbolic communication was almost frighteningly clear and recognizable.

After about six to eight months of working together, Leah began to come out of the corner much earlier every session. In one particular session, she came in and chose her own music. *(The act of a client selecting his/her own music signifies a stage of autonomy development.)* Ganet-Sigel put the record player on. Almost immediately Leah came right up to her and pushed her down on the floor. Ganet-Sigel's heart began palpitating. She wondered what was going to happen and if Leah was going stomp on her face or on her stomach. Although Ganet-Sigel had become quite nervous, she remained quiet. She felt that she needed to trust Leah and believe that she had become bonded to her in some way. Ganet-Sigel decided to go with the flow of the session.

After pushing Ganet-Sigel to the floor, Leah pushed Ganet-Sigel's legs apart and exposed her pelvic region, although Ganet-Sigel remained fully clothed. Suddenly, Ganet-Sigel's blood began to curdle, not from nervousness but from excitement about what might be happening. Leah curled herself into a ball, moved very close to her and then she slithered out, almost like a snake. At this point, Ganet-Sigel's blood began to boil even more. *(Ganet-Sigel withheld her interpretation waiting to be certain that her intuition and clinical knowledge were at least 95% accurate. It is essential that the dance/movement therapist be quite certain that his/her interpretation is accurate before sharing any information with the client.)* So she let Leah's movement continue without interruption. Leah curled herself up again in ball and slithered out of Ganet-Sigel's pelvic region two or three more times.

Suddenly, with the realization of what was happening, Ganet-Sigel, very cautiously, with almost a shimmer in her voice said, "a beautiful little girl is being born to us." *(Ganet-Sigel was careful to say that Leah was being born "to us," and not "to me," because it was not the therapist to whom this experience was happening. It was a symbolic birth or rebirthing.)* Her heart was pounding but she didn't want to move a muscle for fear of spoiling what was happening. At the same time she saw the clock and realized that Leah's session was almost over and that there were other clients to see. (*This is one of the sad sagas of being a therapist. The therapist must keep time going and help patients put closure to their sessions even when they are in the midst of high drama and excitement, as very deep and intense issues emerge.)*

Before repeating that, "a beautiful little girl is being born to us," Leah was told that there was time for one more melody and then the session will have to be over. Despite the fact that Ganet-Sigel kept repeating that it was almost time for the session to close, Leah continued to recurl herself and slither out of the womb. However, almost to the minute, Leah stood up and took the needle off the record player. To Ganet-Sigel's amazement, shock, and excitement, there was a little girl standing before her. No longer did she have her wrist, neck or knees bent, or her head extended from her neck and shoulders as an animal standing on its hind legs. Leah was standing aligned and upright as a beautiful little child. She smiled, walked to the door, opened the door, and waved good-bye to Ganet-Sigel. Although Ganet-Sigel knew she had to follow Leah back to the classroom, she lay on the floor almost paralyzed.

At the end of the day, Ganet-Sigel returned home and began to reflect about the events of this day. She thought about how she had witnessed such an exciting, thrilling symbolic growth in a client. This session was one of the highlights in her career. Would she ever observe such a powerful transformation in other clients? For a moment she began to think that perhaps she should stop her work as a dance-movement therapist. However, the events that had occurred in Leah's session also made her realize the healing potential of dance-movement therapy and reaffirmed her belief that dance-movement therapy was really good work. Sometime after Leah terminated at the nursery school, Ganet-Sigel was apprised that Leah had become quite well integrated into the classroom at a public school and was a model student.

This case illustrates how the therapist established a form of mutual communication and used dance/movement to entice an autistically withdrawn child from a private world into our own. This therapeutic breakthrough exceeds the potential of our usual mode of verbal communication and intervention. Rather than relying upon theoretical models that stress pathology, Ganet-Sigel worked to expand Leah's movement repertoire and accentuate the healthy parts of her. She entered Leah's world by reenacting her movements. By reproducing her gestures and movement, she was able to establish trust and lead Leah to communicate repressed feelings and risk new experiences. In this context, Ganet-Sigel used her body to communicate her acceptance of Leah and to validate Leah's expression.

The dyadic movement interactions between Ganet-Sigel and Leah provided this client with the kinesthetic experience of being lovable and held, thereby providing her with a good enough parent for her inner child. Through the kinesthestic experience of being held, Leah was able to internalize the therapist while the negative parental experiences could be neutralized or diminished.

Ganet-Sigel used parts of Chace's framework for establishing therapeutic goals in her work with Leah. She established several goals related to the therapeutic relationship and the concepts of body action and symbolism. Within the domain of the therapeutic relationship, Ganet-Sigel helped Leah establish her own identity and she fostered trust. Within the domain of body action, she focused the movement towards helping Leah to: (1) reconstruct her postural gestalt, (2) become aware of her body sensations, (3) activate and integrate body parts, and (4) mobilize energy. In relationship to the concept of symbolism, Ganet-Sigel encouraged Leah to expand her symbolic repertoire. The distortions in Leah's body posture and function were indicative of maladaptive responses to conflict. However, as she was able to integrate and feel the action in her body, there was a shift in psychic attitudes. The close relationship between postural changes and psychic attitudes can be realized only when the client is ready and when the feelings become meaningful. Only then will there be a change in body image.

As Ganet-Sigel mirrored Leah's movements, Leah felt affirmation and acceptance. Her patience in letting Leah's own sense of discovery and timing guide the flow of the sessions was eventually integrated by

Leah. Accepting Leah's expression, without judgment, was a cue to Leah that she had been validated. Her use of empathetic movement reflection encouraged the development of a healthy therapeutic symbiotic relationship and paved the way for healthy separation-individuation. The symbiotic mirroring transference provided a foundation for establishing levels of bodily object relations differentiation. First, differentiation of me/not me occurred with the therapist, and then differentiation in relation to Leah's internal and external world took place, and finally a level of differentiation grounded in a conscious reality based on thought and action was illustrated by Leah's rebirth. As Leah's viscera ingested the constancy of love, patience, a holding environment, and good enough mothering, she was able to regard Ganet-Sigel as a significant maternal figure in her life. Initially, she relied on Ganet-Sigel's ego for strength, but gradually, Leah realized enough ego strength to become an autonomous being.

As a novice therapist, Ganet-Sigel reified her belief in the importance of relying upon her own clinical knowledge, intuition, and conviction that all clients strive to achieve health. As a therapist, she also began to fully appreciate the potential of dance/movement therapy as a treatment modality.

CHAPTER 6

The Borderline Personality Disordered Patient: Sylvia

Guiding Questions

1. *In what ways can dance/movement therapy be instrumental in the treatment of a client with borderline personality disorder?*

2. *On a motoric and psychological level, what were Sylvia's presenting problems?*

3. *Why do researchers believe that there is a connection between borderline personality disorder and post-traumatic stress disorder (PTSD)?*

4. *What techniques did Ganet-Sigel use in her therapeutic treatment of Sylvia?*

5. *Why is it important for the therapist to clearly distinguish between empathy and sympathy?*

6. *How did Sylvia's expression of movement change during therapy?*

We might try to retrieve the physical consciousness of unalterable grief aroused in us by Martha Graham's dance "Lamentation," with only feet and hands visible outside draped fabric — and agony expressed through stress lines in the cloth. To see more, to hear more. By such experiences we are not only lurched out of the familiar and taken for granted, but we may also discover new avenues for action. We may experience a sudden sense of new possibilities and thus new beginnings (Greene, cited in Ornstein & Behar-Horenstein, 1999, p. 46).

In this chapter, the successful treatment of a client diagnosed with borderline personality disorder will be discussed. Dance/movement therapy is a particularly effective modality for this pathology. The treatment process deals directly with: (1) repairing ego deficits that result from early childhood developmental crises, (2) integrating internal representations of self and others, and (3) offering a facilitating environment so that the client can experience a visceral sense of wholeness and safety and also develop a realistic view of self and others, and (4) increasing the client's competency in functioning in the world. Dance/movement therapy offers a secure environment for the client to express a multitude of conflictual feelings while being able to receive the affirmation and unconditional love that is essential to becoming an autonomous being. The dance/movement therapist accepts the client despite a transference of intense anger and rageful behaviors, impulsivity, unpredictability among other emotions, and remains a stable support figure who provides object constancy. In the treatment process, the dance/movement therapist provides a safe environment in which the client can sustain a healthy symbiosis, neutralize negative parental introjects, and bring preverbal and/or unconscious psychic wounds to a conscious level.

Several theorists have discussed the developmental origins of the borderline personality disorder (Berelowitz & Tarnopolsky, 1993; The Blancks, 1994; Freed, 1984; Kernberg, 1976; Mahler, 1968, 1975; Masterson, 1981; Schwarz & Perry, 1994; Winnicott, 1965; Wolberg, 1982). With the exception of Berelowitz and Tarnopolsky (1993) and Schwarz and Perry (1994), all of the views described below suggest that the etiology of borderline pathology reflects ego deficits that result from developmental crises. Theorists tend to agree that the borderline personality disorder arises primarily from an inability to fuse representations of the self with parental representations, although they differ in opinion as to the exact onset of these conditions. There is also general agreement that the borderline patient's behavior is characterized by passivity and regression, while the development of the true self becomes blocked. Clinging and distancing become primary defense mechanisms to mitigate the overwhelming feelings of emptiness, loneliness, and depression (Freed, 1984).

Kernberg (1976) has attributed the emergence of the borderline disorder to the child's inability to integrate good and bad self representations sometime between the fourth month of life to the end of the first year in the third stage of development during which normal internalized object relations would occur. During this stage, the child typically begins to differentiate self-representations from his/her object relations. However, in dysfunctional development, the good and bad images of self and object remain separated. Although the mother is perceived as distinct from the self, because of this unresolved developmental crisis, she is viewed as either all good or all bad depending upon her response to the child. She is viewed as all good when she gratifies the child, but is perceived as all bad when she frustrates the child. The defense of splitting develops to protect the child from the loss of the good object and good self.

Even though the child is able to differentiate himself/herself from others, his/her identity does not coalesce. The child's development is arrested, a healthy symbiosis between mother and child does not emerge, and he/she does not go on to the fourth stage in which the good and bad images become integrated. The child's capacity to diffuse aggressive impulses is deficient. Additionally his/her ability to regulate other drives is also impaired. Without having developed a healthy bond with the mother, these developmental deficits compromise the patient's ability to perceive and relate to others in functional and adaptive ways. The behavior of the borderline patient is predictably unstable (Freed, 1984). The patient often exhibits impaired interpersonal relations, mood, and self-image. Several symptoms of the borderline patient include depression, impulsivity, unpredictability, attitude changes, identity confusion, intense anger (rageful behavior), extreme loneliness, and emptiness. Kernberg (1976) also argued that while object relations are always impaired, cognitive and other functioning may not be.

Although he concurred with Kernberg's identification of the development of the borderline patient's early childhood difficulties, Mahler (1975) pointed out that the onset of the development crisis occurs during the rapprochement subphase of the separation-individuation process. Unlike Kernberg, Mahler emphasized that it is the primary caregiver's (mother) emotional unavailability and lack of attunement to the unique characteristics of the child that lead to the inception of the borderline conditions. The mother must support the child's efforts to be autonomous and remain a stable figure that the child can count on and receive affirmation from his/her new achievements. Failure to master the rapprochement phase impairs the child's ability to achieve object constancy. The inability to secure an inner representation of the mother impedes consolidation of the self as well as the child's ability to formulate a realistic view of others.

Although Masterson (1981) also attributed the borderline disorder to an unresolved rapprochement crisis, he has emphasized the importance of an abandonment depression as the etiology of the borderline conditions. This depression results from the mother's withdrawal from the child as he/she tries to be autonomous. However, while the child asserts himself/herself, he/she may simultaneously be rewarded by the mother for exhibiting dependent behavior. The child experiences his/her autonomy behavior as confusion, aloneness and rejection, and simultaneously feels anger, guilt, depression, helplessness, and emptiness. As a result, maladaptive coping mechanisms and defense mechanisms emerge to help ward off painful and often intolerable feelings. Successful movement through subsequent developmental phases thus becomes impaired. Manifestations of the borderline pathology are demonstrated by the patient's self-representations which alternate between brittle, vulnerable, self-depreciative, clinging behaviors, and erratic and irrational outbursts of rage.

Drawing upon Mahler's (1975) work, Gertrude and Rubin Blanck (1994), suggested that the borderline pathology is the result of a developmental arrest during the separation-individuation process. In contradistinction to other theorists, they take a broader view of the origins of the disorder. They claim that there is a range of pathologies within the neurotic and psychotic borders. Arguing that there is more than one type of borderline disorder, they claimed that it is where particular subphase difficulties occur, how they were handled, and how the ego negotiated these challenges that determine the specific manifestations of the borderline pathology.

Winnicott (1965) emphasized the primacy of the environment. He asserted that in order for the child to experience healthy development, he/she must have a facilitating environment in which the primary maternal figure meets the child's needs and relates to the child by providing good enough mothering. This phase represents the major objects relations development of the child's growth. If the child fails to have these needs fulfilled, he/she may develop a false self to adapt to the demands of the mother in order to receive her love and have his/her needs met. These environmental conditions may lead to the development of the borderline conditions.

In an updated review of the validity of research on borderline personality disorder, Berelowitz and Tarnopolsky (1993) discussed etiology of the disorder. They observed that several retrospective studies (Brown & Anderson, 1991; Bryne, Velamoor, & Cernovsky, et al., 1990; Herman, Perry, & Van Der Kolk, 1988; Links, Steiner, & Offord, et al., 1998, Nigg, Silk, & Westen, et al., 1991; Ogata, Silk, & Goodrich, 1990; Zanarini, Gunderson, & Frankenburg, et al., 1989) lend substantial support to the notion that borderline personality disorder emerges from a combination of factors that occur in the childhood environment such as neglect, instability, martial discord, physical and sexual abuse and the absence of a good relationship, primarily with a maternal caregiver, that can buffer the adverse variables present in the environment. Moreover, they claimed that the evidence of a relationship between the development of borderline pathology and a history of childhood sexual and physical abuse and neglect is strong. They questioned the validity of Mahler's (Mahler, Pine, & Bergmann, 1975) theoretical work in which he and his associates suggested that the unresolved rapprochement phase leads to behavior similar to that observed in adult borderline patients. In his work with toddlers aged 18–24 months, a time when infants learn object constancy and the capacity for ambivalence, Mahler et al. (1975) observed that mothers responded to infants with aggression or withdrawal and that subsequently the infants alternated between clingingness and withdrawal.

Schwarz and Perry (1994) suggested that there is a relationship between traumas experienced during childhood and adolescence and the development of the borderline personality disorder. They claimed that children, diagnosed with post-traumatic stress disorder, who are traumatized chronically can also develop symptoms that meet the criteria for borderline personality disorder. PTSD may emerge from malignant memories that coalesce in response to a traumatic stressor. The extent to which an individual experiences an event as traumatic is a function of many factors including, among others, their progression along the developmental trajectory, neuropsychological processes, age, resilience, vulnerability and protective factors. The authors asserted that:

> Malignant memories rooted in early trauma are likely to manifest later as disorders of the self, personality [such as borderline personality disorder], or ego functions including cognitive development and regulation of object relations, attention, affect, and arousal, and are not usually recalled as deriving from discrete events (p. 315).

They have also claimed that there are physiological components common to both disorders. Similar alterations in variety of neuroendocrine and blood element markers have been observed in both the borderline personality disordered and PTSD patients.

Based upon his experiences with borderline patients who have PTSD, Kroll (1997) stated that there appears to be a close correlation between individuals who exhibit disassociative episodes and self-injurious behaviors and severe traumatic experiences such as childhood abuse. He believes that it may be helpful to view such borderline patients as suffering from a chronic form of PSTD in which such symptoms are indicative of an upbringing characterized by toxicity and stress. He suggested that many of the predominate symptoms seen in the PTSD patients such as "intrusive reexperiencing of traumatic events, . . . avoidance of stimuli reminiscent of traumatic events, . . . psychic numbing, . . . increased psychological and physiological arousal" are also exhibited by patients who suffer from the borderline condition with a history of abuse (cited in Rosenbluth, 1997, p. 98).

Understanding the etiology of the borderline conditions is instrumental in helping the therapist: (1) interpret the symptoms and behavior of the borderline patient, (2) formulate expectations about the patient's abilities and limitations, (3) establish treatment goals, and (4) identify appropriate therapeutic interventions. For example, recognizing that the borderline patient is unable to fuse representations of the self with parental representations, the dance therapist creates a therapeutic environment that lends itself to the client's ability to experience a healthy symbiotic bond by providing object constancy, a holding environment, and good enough mothering. By observing the client's movement repertoire, the therapist attunes himself/herself to the client's body language and psychic attitudes. The dance therapist uses this information to establish treatment goals, and select movement techniques that will help the client reveal intrapsychic attitudes and feelings. The therapist may also lend his/her ego to help the client secure an inner representation of the good enough mother, so that his/her identity can coalesce.

The Case of Sylvia

Sylvia, who had been hospitalized for a long period of time without much success, contacted Ganet-Sigel and asked if she could make an appointment. Sylvia explained that she had been referred by one of her dance/movement therapy interns, Mary, and her psychiatrist, Dr. Aaron Russet. Even though Dr. Russet did not know much about dance/movement therapy, he requested that Ganet-Sigel work with Sylvia. Later as a result of Sylvia's progress, Dr. Russet began referring other patients to her and they developed a working relationship. Russet claimed that dance/movement therapy had the capacity ". . . to do things that medication and verbal psychotherapy can't." He believed that dance/movement therapy was ". . . more effective than just verbal psychotherapy and medication management alone."

When Ganet-Sigel and Sylvia initially met, they sat down and talked for just over an hour. During this time, Sylvia discussed how she came to meet Ganet-Sigel and why she wanted to work with a dance/movement therapist. Sylvia explained to Ganet-Sigel that she had recently been released from a psychiatric hospital rather abruptly due to a lack of insurance coverage. At the time of her release, she reported that she was just beginning to deal with some significant traumatic childhood issues during therapeutic work with Ganet-Sigel's intern, Mary. Sylvia recounted that almost immediately, she had became attracted to dance/movement therapy and felt love towards Mary. Sylvia's work with the intern ended prematurely after about one month of working together. Sylvia told Ganet-Sigel that when she first learned about Mary's departure, she felt abandoned. She recounted how shortly after her discharge from the hospital, her feelings of vulnerability, loneliness and fright reached levels that she could not tolerate. In response to her own uneasiness, she told Dr. Russet to find her a dance/movement therapist. Sylvia explained that she instructed him to, "Find me a dance/movement therapist, or you will have one very dead patient on your hands." During their initial meeting, Ganet-Sigel learned that Sylvia was a very angry woman who felt victimized by many people and institutions. She also sensed that Sylvia was a very frightened individual.

Ganet-Sigel offered to work with her at no charge on two conditions; that Sylvia came to each and every session and that she would be able to leave each session on her own two feet. This Ganet-Sigel insisted upon, because there could be no ambulances, medics, or emergency rescue teams coming to save Sylvia if they were going to have an effective "working" relationship. In short, she said, "you have to be able to survive outside the hospital."

Sylvia attended sessions twice a week. By her own account, Sylvia related that she had been quite ill for many years. Over a thirteen year period various psychiatrists had prescribed more than 70 different psychotropic drugs to treat her disorder. During her recent hospitalization, Dr. Russet discovered that she showed signs of kidney failure due to intensive drug therapy. Treatment with medication could no longer serve as viable therapeutic intervention for her. Because of her physical condition, Russet determined that if Sylvia was going to experience any significant healing, the development of a healthy therapeutic relationship was the only appropriate intervention.

When Ganet-Sigel first began seeing her, Sylvia related that she had already had eighteen unsuccessful years of verbal therapy. *(Some verbal therapists lack the skills needed to facilitate the revelation of certain emotional crisis within clients.)* She also stated that she had been raped by a psychologist who was treating her. Sylvia was not in contact with any of her family members. She adamantly explained that she did not want them to know where she was living. At the time Sylvia was living in a group residential home for persons with mental illness and physical handicaps. Fearful of the owners and many of the residents who she stated reminded her of her father, she confessed that she loathed this environment because she had no one with whom she felt she could

relate. Shortly after she had begun to work in dance/movement therapy, she moved into a studio apartment. Her support system consisted
of her psychiatrist, Ganet-Sigel, and a long time friend, Ricardo.

Outside of her therapy sessions, Sylvia had a lot of time to herself.
She reported feeling very lonely and vulnerable. Some of the most difficult times she experienced were during nights and weekends. On
many occasions, she lost the ability to speak in complete sentences,
experienced fugue states, laid on the floor drawn up into a fetal position and drooled. She also inflicted wounds and genitalia abuses upon
herself. *(This type of behavior can be disconcerting to the therapist as
well as the client. However, a lack of insurance benefits required that
Sylvia be able to live outside of the hospital or be committed to a state
facility. The role of dance/movement therapist is to continue work
towards therapeutic goals.)*

During the first year and a half of their therapeutic relationship,
Sylvia spent nearly the entire movement part of her session exhibiting
rageful behaviors. At first Sylvia was unable to regulate her own aggression. Her body carriage and posture also provided much insight into
the way she felt. The rigidity and stiffness in her upper body suggested
that she had stuffed feelings of loneliness and sadness into her stomach,
torso, shoulders, and neck. During movement, it was typical to observe
her moving primarily along the outer perimeter of the room. She avoided the center of the room, as if the interior held some fear for her.
When she happened to move away from the outer edges, she was
observed to quickly scamper out of the center back to a zone of safety.
She also avoided any contact with Ganet-Sigel. When Ganet-Sigel
playfully tried to make contact with her, she would turn around and
run from her. Trying to sustain any type of intimacy seemed to be
repellent. *(Sylvia's body broadcast her conflicts. Her breathing was
shallow and arrhythmic. The way she carried herself suggested that she
was not particularly adaptable or able to exercise choice or make decisions freely. The pronounced tension in her pelvis, chest, and neck were
all symptomatic of the conflicts she felt as well as her pervasive mood.)*

Over time it became clear, that, more than anything, Sylvia craved
the closeness available in the initial mother-child bond. She wanted to
be held, rocked, and soothed, but she didn't know how to ask for tenderness. *(As in typical in borderline patients, there is a sense of confusion regarding how to ask for intimacy. Because of the developmental
wounds, the borderline patient believes that a desire for closeness is tied
to the rejection experienced with the primary maternal figure. The fear
of rejection ignites feelings of abandonment, intense anger, loneliness,
and confusion, leaving the patient too emotionally paralyzed to ask
directly for what he/she would have wanted.)* She would bang her head
and fists on the walls and subsequently would fall into a fugue state.
During these periods she experienced amnesia-like qualities in that she
would remember nothing. She stated that during a fugue she felt as "if
my breathing had stopped." Typically her entry back into conscious
thought began with an explosive behavior which consisted of scream-
ing, thrashing and head-banging that seemed to relieve her tension or

facilitate her reemergence into conscious thought. The fugue states became a coping mechanism during her childhood that seemed to help Sylvia cope with the violence and extreme family dysfunctions that had plagued her early life. *(Fugue states are a form of disassociation that relieved Sylvia from having to experience the intensity of her feelings.)*

Subsequently, exhausted by her own raging, Sylvia would collapse into Ganet-Sigel's arms. Ganet-Sigel would hold and rock her until she nearly fell asleep. Ganet-Sigel would tell Sylvia that everything was alright, and that she was safe. *(Ganet-Sigel provided Sylvia with good enough mothering and a holding environment in which she might be able to experience safety and security. She provided a stable support figure in which Sylvia was able to experience a healthy symbiotic bond with a maternal figure.)* Sylvia had difficulty holding the intensity of her anger and her intense desire to be nurtured simultaneously. As Sylvia worked to dissipate her rageful feelings, Jane helped her rechannel the location of her fury into more adaptive forms of communication and expressions. *(Through this experience, Sylvia began to internalize Ganet-Sigel, thus permitting the negative parental introjects to become neutralized. Through this reparenting phase of treatment, Sylvia was able to integrate the good and bad representations of self and others.)* After about one and half years of being nurtured like an infant, Sylvia became autonomous. She was able to receive and follow directions during the movement.

Ganet-Sigel and Sylvia began to move together in dyad. While sitting on the floor and facing one another they also engaged in primary mother-infant play. Using only their hands at first, they explored each other's face. Next they communicated with solely their feet and toes. Next they sculpted one another, putting each other in a position that they wanted the other one to hold. *(Dance/movement therapy acknowledges the primacy of the body movement in communications and recognizes that it is in this mode that healthy realistic self and object representations are first developed (Lewis, 1986).)*

During the verbal portion of their sessions, Ganet-Sigel listened to Sylvia attentively, and tried to convey a sense of empathy and understanding towards Sylvia through her gestures, eyes and posture. However, she was careful to communicate empathy rather than sympathy. *(The distinction between empathy and sympathy must be clear. Empathy is a therapeutic intervention that can help to build therapeutic alliances and establish trust. Empathy also communicates the therapist's attunement with the client, as well as his/her ability to serve as a vessel and hold the client's feelings. Sympathy, on the other hand, is often felt by some clients to be patronizing and condescending. Such a response may inhibit the client's ability to heal and may also result in the therapist merging with the client's dysfunctional behavior.)* Since Sylvia lacked a significant support system, it was important to help her acquire the ability to survive on her own. Showing her sympathy would not have promoted her willingness to survive or helped her develop more adaptive behaviors.

About two years into their relationship, a significant movement event was revealed that ultimately impacted the direction of their therapeutic work. One day, almost immediately as the movement session began, Sylvia lay down onto the floor, quickly fell into a fugue state and began convulsing. Her entire body shook vigorously. She seemed overcome with terror and desperation. She howled in agony, cried, and quivered. Later during the verbal portion their session, she shared a repressed flashback that had plagued her for nearly 28 years. In their session, Sylvia had relived the episode at age 3 1/2 in which she experienced her father "take the dignity and humanity from her sexually," as she "helplessly laid clutched under his bear-like body." Sylvia recounted to Ganet-Sigel, how after the abuse she laid numb with pain and disbelief while she helplessly watched her father turn away to go and find her sister and inflict the same heinous act upon her. Sylvia said that "I felt a terrible deep sadness in my body, but because I lacked the words to express what I had experienced, his unforgivable act became buried. However, my body reminded me to be on guard from that moment forward. I never experienced a peaceful night of sleep in my home throughout my childhood and teenage years while we lived under the same roof. I remained vigilant so I could protect myself."

In subsequent sessions, after the revelation of sexual abuse, Sylvia reported feeling a sudden rush of energy and renewal in her pelvis and her neck from a previously bound up musculature. As a result of this revelation and catharsis, she no longer shunned talking and relating to men or wondered why she had tried so hard to avoid physical intimacy. She shared with Ganet-Sigel that she was no longer curious why she had such difficulty in social interactions with men. She was able to talk about her feelings and the physical somatizations she experienced. She was also able to understand how emotionally arrested she had been become because of the sexual abuse. *(Individuals have the capacity to represent cognitive processes or what they know through memories stored in the perceptual-motor constructs. The continuum of cognitive representations include enactive cognition, iconic cognition, and abstract cognition. Enactive cognition involves "the capacity to remember and reproduce behaviors through the use of physical perceptions of the movement as cues" (Lewis, 1986, p. 223). One of the most basic principles of dance/movement therapy is the recognition of enactive cognition and representation as the most fundamental level of organizing and integrating early developmental phases. Iconic cognition "involves the ability to experience, remember, and reproduce" behavior through the use of imagery, or a series of images as cues (Lewis, 1986, p. 223). Abstract cognition "involves the ability to remember and reproduce" behaviors through the use of concepts, such as written or verbalized words (Lewis, 1986, p. 223). The clients' preferred representative level offers the therapist insight into their cognitive ability. This information can help the therapist discern what is the developmentally appropriate integrative therapeutic process for each client. By acknowledging the status of the client's cognitive capacity, the therapist can also assist him/her in integrating higher forms of representation. Understanding why some clients represent memories via enactive cognition can help explain why verbal therapy may be insufficient for the revelation of an experience that occurred during the preverbal months, even though the memory can be held in the body (Lewis, 1986, p. 223). Once the repressed memory of sexual abuse was revealed and Sylvia had visual memories, she was able to work more consciously on her issues, making the connections between her movement, behavior, and feelings.)*

As their bond of trust matured, Sylvia was able to make significant progress in remediating early childhood developmental crises. For example, when Sylvia was able to get directly angry at Ganet-Sigel, have her anger heard and not experience abandonment, the frequency of her fugue states lessened.

Ganet-Sigel worked with Sylvia to formulate a realistic image of her body by encouraging her to begin to move parts of her body that were stiffened. She also helped her to focus on aligning her body, to become more aware of her visceral sensations, and to mobilize an adaptive use of her energy through breathing exercises and directed movement. Ganet-Sigel worked with Sylvia to integrate her words, experiences, and actions, to externalize thoughts and feelings rather than somatize. She encouraged Sylvia to resolve conflicts as she gained insight and to make explicit behavioral changes by trying new behaviors in social situations. *(Over time, Ganet-Sigel helped Sylvia establish her own identity, develop trust in their relationship, become more independent, and begin to create a healthy social awareness.)*

Sylvia's innate capacity for tenacity and survival provided the foundation for their therapeutic alliance. Sylvia was able to stay in dance/movement therapy and allow herself to be reparented through their relationship. This process was one of the therapeutic interventions that helped Sylvia make the kind of behavioral and interpersonal changes that paved the way for stability and recovery.

Seven and half years into their work, Sylvia was offered a new job in another state. During her final session, she stated that she had integrated Ganet-Sigel's presence in her body, speech, and behavior. Sylvia also shared that her ability to feel Ganet-Sigel 's tenderness and warmth was a primary impetus for helping her move forward to a new phase of life. As they parted and shared a tearful good-bye, Sylvia left Ganet-Sigel with the following poem.

Ode to a New Life

Many years ago I thrust upon your doorstep
    shattered and maligned
    timorously and ungraciously,
Offering the refuse of my being.
    And with tenacity you breathed life into the corpse
        of a shadowy image.
    You transmuted love
        and
    while mending the corpuscles
    strewn amidst the fragments
        you threaded hope.

Despite the shrieks
   that echoed timpanic agony,
      your pulsating gestures
      rewrote the cadence.
Having internalized a softer
   pallet, the luminous vibration
      sings
   a grand pause.
Now followed by a mellow
   rubato,
      the rhythm meters quietly
   softly embracing the warm tenderness
   and love nestled within.
Nestled in the bosom of your arms,
   I learned to know the feeling of being unified like one soul.
Softness and visceral acceptance
   touched the void.
   And while the emptiness washed away,
      a soothingness began
   to hold the weeping muscles.
Time and process
   permitted a felt internalization.
Now tears speak fear
   the womb of replenishment still beckons.
Pushing and pulling,
   as my body struggles to balance.
A trembling gnaw threatens to close the system.
   But, the touch stays,
      the bonding never lost,
         only rekindled
         and recreated.
Dreams of an undignified journey.
   Ghost of a memory past.
   Longing and lacking,
I now hold both terror and joy.
Weeping tissues
   inspire a gnawing void.
Thrusting, flowing, floating
   yield a metric pulsating
Although seemingly carried on wings of angels
I steadfastly steer all the while.

Today Sylvia is living a happy and productive life.

CHAPTER 7

The Anorexia Nervosa Patient: Cassie

Contributors: *Barbara Cargill, Jane Ganet-Sigel, and Linda S. Behar-Horenstein*

Guiding Questions

1. *In what ways can dance/movement therapy be instrumental in the treatment of a client with anorexia nervosa?*

2. *What are the psychological and physical issues that comprise this disease?*

3. *On a motoric and psychological level, what were Cassie's presenting problems?*

4. *How did Cassie's family influence her recovery?*

5. *What techniques did Ganet-Sigel use in her therapeutic treatment of Cassie?*

6. *How did Cassie's expression of movement change during therapy?*

7. *How does the body language of a patient guide the therapist?*

So movement evidently reveals many different things. It is the result of the striving after an object deemed valuable, or a state of mind. Its shapes and rhythms show the moving person's attitude in a particular situation. It can characterize momentary mood and reaction as well as constant features of personality. Movement may be influenced by the environment of the mover (Laban, 1971, p. 2).

This chapter will focus on the treatment of anorexia nervosa through methods of dance/movement therapy. An example drawn from a successfully treated case is used to share how dance/movement therapy is an effective treatment modality for this pathology. Dance/movement therapy deals directly with the formation of a realistic body image, the recapitulation of missed developmental stages (Krueger & Schofield, 1986), and the provision of opportunities for the anorexic to experience a felt sense of body and the cognitive connections leading to integration and individuation.

Dance/movement therapy, as a body centered therapy, is especially powerful with an anorexic since it provides a potent yet gentle atmosphere for trust and bonding. Through the powerful interventions that movement offers, the anorexic patient has the opportunity to repair the preverbal as well as the present wounds. The dance therapist is an ally of both the inner child and the emerging adult and supports the full-bodied life. The treatment is a journey of discovery, trading addiction for spontaneity and exchanging a mechanical goal-oriented life for a creative life fully grounded in the body.

Anorexia nervosa is a multi-faceted psychosomatic disorder characterized by self-starvation. In this disorder a deep sense of unworthiness pervades the life of the victim leading to a striving for perfection. The anorexic compensates for overwhelming feelings of grief and abandonment with an excessive need for control eventually leading to weight control. The compulsive attitude towards weight and food overshadows his or her whole life. The family appears close knit and loving, seems to "deal" with the patient and describes the victim as a "good girl" before the disease onset. However, in actuality she is a symptom bearer for a complex family pathology (Minuchin, Rosman, & Baker, 1978).

Anorexics are primarily adolescent girls (10% are males). They are usually from middle class affluent families. The onset occurs frequently at pubescence or at 18 when the child leaves home for the first time; both times are "rites of passage." The psychological symptoms of anorexia include: a marked distortion of body image, concrete thinking that is devoid of imagination, a relentless pursuit of thinness, a drive for control and attention, hyperactivity, and chronic deep-seated depression. There is a denial of any bodily symptoms including hunger and fatigue and a denial of the fact that a problem even exists. The perfection issues, including over-achievement and compulsive behavior toward food, exercise, and activities, are attempts to have absolute control over an out-of-control life and serve to keep the anorexic too busy to experience the extreme underlying anxiety, rage, and despair. According to Krueger and Schofield (1986), since clients with anorexia nervosa have never initially integrated mind and body, they lack the capacity to defensively split body awareness and feelings. Because they lack a consolidated body image and have a nuclear formation of self that is disorganized and primitive, anorexics suffer from an inability to recognize and distinguish among different affects and bodily sensations.

The pressure of our highly technological society for achievement, affluence, and thinness impacts the prevalence of this pathology. In contrast, it has been observed that countries in which there is not enough food have little or no incidence of anorexia. Open any Western teen magazine and you will see skeletal, airbrushed models in designer clothing; recipes for high calorie desserts opposite diet plans, and all the latest exercise fads for teens. Media depictions offer role confusion for many women. Having too many choices and being expected to launch a professional career while still being a perfect mother impacts many, if not most, women. In addition, all eating disorders are often symptomatic of other underlying childhood trauma such as childhood sexual abuse (Blume, 1990).

The physical diagnosis of anorexia is based on a loss of over 25% of body weight, hyperactivity, hypothermia, a growth of fine hair over the body and delay of, or cessation of menses. Minuchin et al., (1978) report that 25% of anorexics have bulimia (binge and purge syndrome). Anorexia nervosa has a 10–15% mortality rate (Minuchin et al., 1978). Ideally anorexia is treated using a combination of approaches including close medical supervision, family therapy, individual and group therapy, and from these authors' experiences, treatment based on the principles of dance/movement therapy.

The dance/movement therapist formulates treatment goals based on the individual's needs. Some of the tools dance therapists use are rhythmic activities, kinesthetic empathy, intentional touch, visual imagery, relaxation techniques, mirroring, art and movement combinations, use of transitional objects, body-image work, dream work, music, guided imagery, improvisational movement with music, verbal therapy, and breath work. Bioenergetics, yoga, psychodrama, and other techniques are also very useful.

In anorexia there is a severe distortion of body image. The body image is a combination of the idea/picture that one has of one's body and the sensate experience of the body. The body image is formed in early life by the kinesthetic experiences in infancy which leave impressions on the brain (Lowen, 1967). Articulation of body parts, recognition and satiation of body sensation, awareness of muscular activity, and, most importantly, the quality of nurturing and touch between the infant and primary care figure all contribute to the formation of body image. This original infant/mother symbiosis can be reconstructed through the non-verbal interaction between patient and therapist in dance/movement therapy and slowly change the body image to a more positive one. Marion Chace, the founder of dance/movement therapy, states, "Since motion influences body image and psychic attitude then if you can work a feeling of distortion of body image out in motion you can change your psychic attitude toward yourself" (Chaiklin, 1984, p. 228). Thus body image work is an integral part of the treatment plan for anorexia.

The client's movement bears the imprint of the past and reveals a person's past conscious and unconscious experience. The dance therapist is a skilled observer of body language and the dynamics of movement and uses these skills for diagnosis and intervention. Movement crystallizes and integrates the physiological and psychological. This will be illustrated by the following case study.

The Case of Cassie

Cassie, a 16 year old woman, called to make an appointment with Ganet-Sigel. During the first session she proceeded to tell Ganet-Sigel that she attempted suicide about six months previously, and had wanted to die since the age of ten. She felt guilty about everything, and she was unhappy about her situation at home. Her mother and father had been divorced for five years; her father was remarried for three years. She had a natural sister, seventeen, and stepsisters who were eleven and nine. She hated her new stepmother. Prior to her suicide attempt she was in a psychiatric hospital for six weeks. Afterwards she was in verbal therapy for a short time (6 months). She consistently got more anxious, was getting progressively thinner by starving herself, and was alternately throwing up and bingeing. When she started therapy with Ganet-Sigel, a physical examination by a physician was ordered. The medical problems involved in throwing up and dieting were discussed. Ganet-Sigel made it clear to her, after explaining all of the physiological and psychological connections, that if she reached a certain loss of body weight that that she would have to be hospitalized.

The medical examination revealed little damage to her physical health at this point. She was 98 pounds, although in the next couple of months she went down into the upper 80's. She was extremely hyperactive, had a growth of fine hair all over her body, and had not menstruated in two years. She had compulsive fetishes toward her food, walked dozens of miles a day, and was preoccupied with her "fat stomach" in the mirror. She was angry and alternately depressed. She hated her father, her stepmother, and her mother.

Early in the therapeutic alliance, Ganet-Sigel saw her family, both individually and jointly. There was a real deprivation of love and lack of desire for this child. The father married out of guilt. The parents were at odds throughout their relationship. The natural mother, despondent and depressed most of the time, was unable to take care of Cassie in an adequate manner. The first child was acting up, causing the mother a lot of concern and the second child, Cassie, was described as no real problem. Her mother reported she was always good, quiet, and well-behaved. Later it was revealed in Cassie's therapy that she felt she had to please both mother and father; however, nothing seemed to satisfy them. This family did not permit Cassie to express her own individuality. Cassie received a lot of material giving but not the giving of interpsychic love, consistency, and limits that she needed all along. Cassie said that there was "no one in the whole wide world that she could trust," and that "everything always went wrong when she tried to do something good."

The beginning goal for therapy was to develop trust, foster a feeling of autonomy, form a realistic self-image, and build a healthy body concept. In the beginning phase of therapy, which Ganet-Sigel calls the "regurgitation period," Cassie was encouraged to talk as freely, as comfortably and openly as she wanted to. She moved around the room if she wanted to, sat where she wanted, and asked as many questions of Ganet-Sigel as she wanted. She was very concerned if Ganet-Sigel had ever worked with people like her before, concerned that she was all by herself, different, a freak, and weird. She needed to have a validation of her sameness during almost every session.

Although Cassie was a very beautiful young woman, with auburn hair and expressive hands and body, there was a marked distortion of how she saw herself. She wore long-sleeved heavy sweaters, and over that usually a loose-fitted, wide shirt or blouse, very baggy pants, large jeans or overalls, and boots. Clothing hid her body and if she could have covered her face and not be seen, she probably would have. Although weight was a very crucial part of Cassie's present problem, Ganet-Sigel's opinion was that she did not want to focus on the weight and the malnutrition, but on the underlying features of the problem. Ganet-Sigel believed that the diminished weight was just a symptom of Cassie's illness. Cassie talked about her weight, her throwing up, her eating habits. She was very well-versed about the number of calories in everything from a leaf of lettuce to a dish of pasta.

Ganet-Sigel tried to get support from the parents, but there was conscious and unconscious sabotage of the therapy. The family professed to be interested and caring but never came in for regular sessions. They would come in intermittently for a session or two. Because of this situation, the best that could be done was to strengthen Cassie's healthy manifestations, diminish the symptoms that produced rage and despondency, and strengthen her autonomy. The issues of autonomy and trust were initially addressed by having Cassie choose her own record. She would come in for weeks and say "no, you choose the record, you know best," (a behavior that was typical of the way she sacrificed her individuality to parents, peers, society). Ganet-Sigel gently insisted that she choose her own record, that her choice was good, no matter what it was, that there was no good or bad, right or wrong, that what she did was hers and what she did was all right. For many months, if there was a record left on the record player from the previous session, Cassie would look at it and say, "Oh, this looks like a good one, let's use this one." At least this was a start. Although it was not her own choice, at least she thought that it was. Over time, Cassie was able to develop the capacity to form a definite opinion about what she wanted to dance to. In the beginning, she turned off music with sexual overtones. At first, Ganet-Sigel guided the warm-ups for her. *(This was to help her begin to focus on different areas of her body and to develop the felt sense of body parts necessary to awaken body image reformation.)* She responded to outer directions at this time in her life more easily than her own inner direction. Although she needed to be autonomous, she also needed to be encouraged to get in touch with her body in different ways. Gradually the warm-ups became her own.

She would listen to and feel her head and the way it moved, and then move slowly down through the body, to arms, shoulders, chest, her breathing, wrists, fingers, stomach, hips, genitalia, buttocks, back, thighs, ankles, calves, and feet. *(Not only did this process give Cassie an opportunity to get in touch with every part of her body, but it also gave Ganet-Sigel a way to look at her movement diagnostically.)* As she went through different parts of her body, Ganet-Sigel was able to observe which parts she was resistant to move, the rigidity, fear, fluidity, calmness, the obsessional movements, the repetition in movements, her rhythm, force, timing, and how she used her body in space. These observations provided therapeutic clues about what her body was saying. Her improvisations at the end of the guided warm-ups were limited and sometimes erratic. Occasionally, she would be tremendously explosive in her entire body and yet narrow in her use of space. Cassie spent a lot of time on the floor. During many sessions, she just moved into fetal positions, and remained rigid, bound, and fearful of standing on her feet. Cassie worked hard at remaining a child. Developmentally she was arrested in an infantile stage.

She had many aching needs that not been met. Her mother had said Cassie rarely had to be held, rocked, touched. In their sessions, Cassie was extremely needy of touching and nurturing. She did a lot of nurturing of herself in the fetal position. Ganet-Sigel did very little intervening or moving with Cassie in the first phase of the therapeutic work for several reasons. Although Cassie was very needful of touching and tactile stimulation and although she was doing a lot of self-stimulating, she was also very fearful of this touching from anyone else. *(Ganet-Sigel believed that Cassie needed to develop more trust in the therapeutic alliance, and of the whole movement process, without judgment or interference. Cassie needed to move as she felt. The body image techniques, the directed warm-ups, and the expressive movement gave her a chance to explore her own boundaries and rhythms and sense her body in her own way without any judgment put upon her and her movement patterns.)* When they entered into the verbal part of the therapy, they would talk about Cassie's feelings, what was happening, and what was emerging. Their conversations about what was emerging were eventually used to build future movement sessions.

Cassie began to enjoy her own space. She would verbalize, "I like having my own space." This was the early stage of individuation, of the differentiation from father and mother. She liked not having to prove herself to someone else. She spent a lot of time touching herself, being tactile with things in the room, making object relationships, and differentiating herself from a dysfunctional symbiosis of trying to prove herself to her parents. Cassie began to relax as the weeks went on. The use of more body-directed image techniques lead her to feel and experience her body. For example, when Ganet-Sigel used a technique called "isolating body parts," Ganet-Sigel would ask her to let her head lead her movement, and let everything else follow along. Her head was the director. They would later move every part of her body, "Let your arms be the director, let your stomach be the director, let your back, your legs, etc." *(These movement techniques represented the kinds of issues that Cassie was dealing with and also evoked emotional content symbolically.)* She revealed that her head was being directed by her father. She was completely unable to have any freedom in her pelvic area. She was afraid of the sensual and sexual feelings that would come from using this part of her body, and she mentioned many times that she only liked being a little girl.

Cassie gradually became comfortable with the room, but the space between Ganet-Sigel and her was quite apparent. Ganet-Sigel moved her body on a minimal basis, along with Cassie as she was moving, but making no direct connection with her. *(Her movement was purposeful so there was some kinesthetic and visceral acknowledgment that there was another person in the room, but Ganet-Sigel was careful to make no demands on her or hamper her grasping and searching and tentative kinds of reaching out movements that she was looking for to discover the nurturing that was lacking from her past.)* Yet, the fear that she felt was also quite apparent in her eyes. Ganet-Sigel sensed Cassie's fear also from her movement in which she pulled away with her body, shrinking and staying on the floor. However, Ganet-Sigel felt that she needed to wait for Cassie's own timing. Meanwhile they continued to work on increasing her movement repertoire so that she might begin to use her body in many different movements.

They worked with the words *twist, bend, stretch, swing, bounce, shake, push, pull, dodge,* and *strike.* Often Ganet-Sigel would shout out these words during a session, one or two or three a week and repeat each one over a period of time, while there was still no touching. Each one of these words stored up symbolic representations of many things for Cassie. Her movements were alternately still bound, rigid, controlled, and fragmented at times. She used her hands a lot, which were extremely expressive, in contrast to her face and its affect which rarely changed. She twisted with a tremendous amount of energy. In her twisting she began to let go of some of the bound expression in her face. Her stretching was strong, yet her stretching was bound. She did not allow every part of her body to stretch to the fullest extent. She would stretch her arms and a little bit of her legs but not her torso. Bending was easy, as she would bend into her fetal position and then to the floor and stay on the floor. Swing was controlled. Cassie was able to shake herself into a frenzy. Later she stated that *shake* was easy, *twist* was easy, because those were the feelings she experienced most of the time. Cassie felt that she was twisted and distorted in many areas of life. *Swing* was the most difficult thing that she could do. Cassie was afraid of *push* and *pull,* which is what she most wanted to do. She dodged from everything and her striking out was controlled and fearful.

As Ganet-Sigel repeated these words during subsequent sessions, it became apparent that Cassie was opening her repertoire of movement and finding new avenues and awareness. As she worked towards helping Cassie experience releasing and revealing trapped feelings and learning more about her movement, Cassie began to crystallize what she was feeling. Three months into therapy, Cassie seemed a bit more relaxed and anxiously looked forward to coming to sessions. Her questions about whether or not she was weird or strange had ceased. She seemed to want very much to be in the therapy room. At the end of a three-month period, they were able to make their first bodily contact. Cassie allowed Ganet-Sigel to put her hand on her shoulder as she left a session. As Ganet-Sigel told her that she was looking forward to seeing her the next session, Cassie neither pulled her shoulder in or caved in her chest; instead, she gave a genuine smile.

During the next session, Ganet-Sigel began moving into regressional developmental movement patterns, during which she became more actively tactile, touching, and nurturing. Cassie was able to enjoy and have fun with their first mirroring experience. *(Mirroring is a way of exchanging movements in synchrony, where a client and a therapist mirror the movements of each other. Many things can happen through this technique. First of all, the synchrony with which the client and therapist engage can recapitulate the early symbiotic relationship between mother and child.)* The healthy symbiosis that needs to happen before and during individuation and separateness from oneness with Mother was being reenacted this time with an accepting, supportive, primary, nurturing figure. *(Mirroring can also give a client the safety, security, confidence, and self-esteem of seeing someone else reflecting her movements. The client gains an awareness of herself and what her movements are really like.)* The realization that someone else is doing her movements can at first be shocking but also reassuring, nurturing, and affirming of her body image.

This technique can also allow the therapist to introduce new movements, behaviors, and qualities into the client's movement repertoire in order to allow a kinesthetic empathy to develop within the client's body. The therapist can then exaggerate movements of the client, slightly at first, then expanding. This exaggeration into new movements allows the whole visceral sense to come alive. Cassie began to experience an excitement about the synchrony that began to happen over a period of weeks in their mirroring sessions. When synchrony occurs, it is as if the movement happens spontaneously and has its own energy, a revelation to anorexics whose movement and life allows no spontaneity. Trust was beginning to develop. From the synchrony of mirroring, they moved into an exercise of moving into intimate space, but not actually touching yet. An exercise called "statue" was used. *("Statue" is a technique in which the person becomes a statue by holding themselves still, and the other person, without touching them, moves in as close into the intimate space of the other person as possible, exploring that space around them without touching them, exploring the space around all parts of the body, and eventually becomes a statue in that person's space.)* Ganet-Sigel and Cassie did this back and forth alternately.

In the beginning, Cassie never got in front of Ganet-Sigel; she explored her back. She was cautious but creative with her body. She was beginning to use all parts of her body to explore Ganet-Sigel's intimate space. Apparently loving it, she never gave up her role of explorer. She was almost like a child exploring her mother for the first time, but during the verbal processing of their sessions all that she revealed was her wish for the cuddling her mother never gave her. Cassie was giving clues marking the desire for intimacy, trust, and nurturing. Very slowly, they began to going into exercises that could develop into some tactile nurturing. The first exercise was to move through the room together and very slowly touch backs. *(The back is very safe. It is not sexual or particularly sensuous, and no eye contact is involved. The back exercise provided a safe means for the first contact in movement that Cassie and Ganet-Sigel made together.)* All Ganet-Sigel said was, "Talk to me with your back." Cassie was extremely creative. Cassie's body was extremely needful and forceful but resisted receiving. *(While there was a tremendous desire to be given to, she could not yet allow herself (again the ambivalence of trust) to receive the type of tenderness and nurturance she craved.)* They moved from touching and communicating back to back to communicating with just their feet. Next they moved to communicating with their hands, and then gradually they moved to exploring faces, where Ganet-Sigel explored Cassie's face with her hands, and Cassie explored Ganet-Sigel's face with her hands. Subsequently they moved from exploring hands to exploring arms.

Then for the first time, Cassie experienced emotional catharsis and cried. This was the first time that she allowed Ganet-Sigel to nurture and hold her in her arms. As though she were an infant child, Ganet-Sigel rocked her without any words. Cassie was relieved; she had released a tremendous amount of sadness and despondency. She allowed herself to be nurtured, and she especially enjoyed that. From that time on, Cassie had made her transference to Ganet-Sigel. Basic trust was reinforced, and the therapeutic alliance was established.

An explanation of the clinical and theoretical reasons for the slow development of therapeutic alliance, the bonding that took place via body movement between therapist and patient, and the trust issues unique to treating anorexics follows. Treating anorexia has differences in emphasis but not in content from the treatment of other disorders using dance movement therapy. The therapeutic alliance is slow to form. Maintaining trust is the key. Movement is powerful and may bring up emotion quickly of which anorexics are very fearful. One must introduce body work and movement gently with respect for the defenses which protect the fragile sense of self and the hurt child within the anorexic. The pacing must be slow in recognition that patient bonding is very tentative, resulting from an entrenched denial system that serves as a protection for the overwhelming feelings of helplessness and unworthiness. Defenses are respected and befriended, and their manifestations in body structure and movement (e.g. in anorexia the rigid, bound, mechanical, highly controlled, dead affect, and tight musculature) are mirrored until hints of free flow and spontaneity, however small, emerge. The therapist may then use kinesthetic empathy to gently expand the patient's movement repertoire, offering new possibilities which in the safe environment are picked up by the patient creating a synchrony which recalls early child development issues. The therapist continuously empties herself of expectations, by becoming a "good enough surrogate-mother-healer" and "tries to heal" (or keep alive) this difficult and fragile patient.

Dance/movement therapy adds a dimension of play and spontaneity to the treatment of anorexia which decreases the client's defensiveness. The body awareness work, the emotional and sensate connections, the body image work and the playful interaction of "being without doing" experiences in the dance/movement therapy sessions are distinctly missing from the anorexic's existence. Accessing the anorexic's creative force and her authentic movement is a beginning for her to feel the deep sense of loss, loneliness, self-hatred, and rage and later claim her personal power and individuation and to play in the moment of life. The nonverbal interaction between dance/movement therapist and client allows the critical preverbal arrests to be experienced in a kinesthetically healthy symbiosis, leading toward separation and individuation. Cognitive connections are explored constantly as this therapy works at the mind-body interface. When an anorexic can begin to accept her feelings and her body and accept the imperfect human condition, she learns to value herself without having to achieve anything. The emergence into autonomy and the "dance of life" is full-bodied and in flux, unfolding in a metamorphosis that values at a deep level the full-feeling human condition.

Much faith in the method is needed by the therapist when dealing with anorexia, a faith that the intervention appropriate to the moment will be available. *(Dance/movement therapists are well versed in letting go of agendas and capturing the movement as they have come from backgrounds that include improvisational movement.)* The therapy becomes a living energetic unfolding, so unlike the pathology, where life is goal-oriented, categorized, and lived in lists and complex plans. "What wants to happen next" is a metaphor for allowing the healing process to be moved out of the arena of control, stimulating the "inner healer" of the patient and removing the therapist from the position of precarious, outside authority. Stuck places begin to melt without confrontation. The therapist is guide, reflector, and friend of "the patient in his/her entirety."

Very little interpretation is needed as cognitive integration happens throughout the treatment in a natural way once the body messages are clear and the therapeutic alliance is solid. The reconstruction of early developmental gaps by movement interventions, especially mirroring authentic movement, helps insights erupt spontaneously. The freedom to choose new options and become more expressive is a natural evolution. This is a direct result of the body image work, the nonverbal bonding, and the gentle shaking of the rigid body structure through movement and play. The accompanying disorders, the anxiety and dichotomous "all or nothing" thinking (so characteristic of anorexia) can be verbalized and acted out, put into movement, drama, drawings and expressed in the dance/movement therapy treatment room and brought to consciousness. The compulsions, the fears, and the hyperactivity all become part of the dance and are absorbed over time into the energy of the new dyad formed with safety and unconditional love. There is no right or wrong or good or bad as long as physical safety is maintained.

Respect for spatial boundaries is needed when treating this disorder. Anorexics tend to be sensitive to boundaries and experience them as enmeshed, diffused, and constantly invaded. The body language of the patient guides the therapist in making decisions around personal space and timing.

Since, unlike most other psychological disorders, anorexia can be a life/death issue, consistent medical and nutritional management is a necessity. The therapist must keep in mind that when body weight is 25% below normal, the psychological disorientation which can result makes depth therapy difficult if not impossible; and movement may be contraindicated for medical needs. During this crisis the unconditional acceptance and support of the therapist can be very effective. Meth-

ods that are quiet and relaxing are helpful and can foster body awareness and teach the patient to listen to the wisdom of the body.

Relapses are common even when therapy seems to be going well,
as anorexics will comply with rules and regulations to get their own way
and stay in control. This compliant, manipulative "pleasing" behavior
may fool the therapist into believing that progress has been made, and
the therapist must be alert to this behavior and address the feeling component behind it as well as assure the patient that she does not need to
do anything to please her therapist, she is valued just the way she is.
The manipulative behavior and constant relapses can be very disheart-
ening to the therapist and contributes to therapist burn-out when
working with this population.

Countertransference and burn-out are pitfalls when working with
this disorder more often than in most other pathologies. Therapists
may find themselves trapped in the very system they are helping the
client to move out of, e.g., finding oneself working too hard, overpro-
tecting the client in sessions with the family, becoming enmeshed and
triangulated between client and parent and other clinicians and, in general, becoming exhausted and frustrated with the slowness and rigidity
in the process (Bruch, 1978). It is important to keep one's sense of
humor and be a role model for a more playful, positive attitude (Bruch,
1978). Starvation by choice is a serious business, but the cure lies some-
where in the realm of spontaneity and play. When finding oneself stuck
in the client's system, the therapist's honest awareness of her/his own
imperfections and laughable mistakes are a great relief to a client
trapped in the dry desert of perfectionism (Bruch, 1978).

Emotional nourishment must be given at appropriate times and
proportioned according to the person's ability to take it in. You do not
give a shrunken stomach a gourmet meal. Emotional nourishment falls
on deaf ears with anorexics unless the timing is right, only giving it in
moments when it can be received. Addressing what she notices that
prevents the patient from taking in nourishment and encouraging the
patient to study her experience is very helpful in engaging the whole
self to observe split off parts and introjected parental voices. Meditation
techniques[9] that foster the stilling of mental chatter are helpful in treating this disorder. Those techniques that are body centered or those that
give the practitioner something "to do" are preferred over techniques
that focus on emptying the mind or concentrating on an affirmation or
a mantra. Mindfulness is one such method (Kurtz, 1990). In mindfulness, one witnesses and labels one's experience as non-judgments. One
can learn to interact with, and then watch, the internal judgments
rather than react and act from them.

In anorexia, many more body image techniques are used than in
other disorders. The distortion in body image is a core issue and techniques such as body tracings, movement work related to feelings

---

[9] Mindfulness or Vipassana Meditation is a meditation technique 5000 years old. It is
practiced in Buddhist contemplative methods. A modification of Mindfulness is
used in the Hakomi Body Centered Psychotherapy Method. (See Kurtz, 1990).

around body parts, body centered relaxation, isolation of body parts and felt sense movement from those body parts, connective movement from the body core to the joints and appendages, rhythm on body parts, and body sculpting are a few of the many body image techniques dance therapists use.

From this vignette, the reader may become aware that working with anorexia can be an unusually serious responsibility for a therapist. Literally life and death are at stake. A combination of solid medical management with a warm, supportive primary therapist is essential. Body image distortion and psychosomatic symptoms are a core of the disorder, and dance/movement therapy works on both psyche and soma. Dance/movement therapy can greatly accelerate the progress of the client.

Considering the 10–15% death rate among anorexics, it becomes clear that in anorexia some creative methods of approach are desperately needed (Minuchin et al. 1978). From the observations of anorexics and their families, it appears that the normal infant-mother symbiosis was profoundly disturbed. Without the healthy completion of this stage, the infant/adolescent/adult cannot experience the stage of spontaneous play, of "being" without "doing." They engage in dichotomous thinking and do not form healthy relations. Societal pressures for achievement and thinness add to the disorder.

Anorexics are typically "scapegoats" for family pathology and probably never experienced the deep satisfaction of being valued just for their "being" as infants, children or adolescents. Because of the nonverbal emphasis and energy exchanges which occur in dance/movement therapy, this body-centered modality can provide the silent nurturing, the affirmation of body and self, and the recapitulation of the critical pre-verbal kinesthetic experiences so necessary for emotional health, in an atmosphere of unconditional acceptance of body and mind.

Family therapy, in addition to body work and medical management, greatly enhances the success of the treatment. However, families of anorexics can be manipulative, denying, enmeshed and rigid and may actively sabotage therapy. Consistently and predictably, they often avoid taking responsibility for their part in the disorder. In the case of an uncooperative family, it is even more essential to include dance/movement therapy in the treatment plan to help the patient contact and define her bodily existence as separate and unique. Additionally, families need to be informed over and over again that anorexia is a family disease. The mutual cooperation of hospital staff, physicians and therapists is crucial.

As of this writing, Cassie has maintained her weight at a healthy level for several years and feels good about her body and likes being a woman. She becomes bulimic on occasion but recognizes the bulimia as a symptom of buried feelings and is able to process them herself. Her anorexic sister recently entered therapy with Jane Ganet-Sigel.

PART III

A Comparison of *D*ance/ *M*ovement and *V*erbal *P*sychotherapy

Introduction

In chapter eight, the authors compare dance/movement therapy to verbal psychotherapy. They describe dance-movement therapy as a healing modality in its own right and analyze the methodological and philosophical differences between dance/movement and verbal forms of psychotherapy. They also describe the kinesthetic and unconscious processes of dance/movement therapy. Next the authors discuss the interrelationships between kinesthestic and verbal components of dance/movement therapy. Finally they explore why movement interventions permit patients to experience a recovery that is sometimes beyond the realm of strictly verbal interventions.

CHAPTER 8

Dance/Movement Therapy and Verbal Psychotherapy

Guiding Questions

1. According to the authors, what are the goals of dance/movement therapy?

2. How do studies of effectiveness and efficacy differ?

3. What is meta-analysis?

4. Based upon the studies reported in this chapter, how would you characterize the effectiveness of dance/movement therapy?

5. How has dance/movement therapy been used in working with various patient populations?

6. In what ways does dance/movement therapy differ from strictly verbal forms of psychotherapy?

If psychoanalysis brings about a change in the mental attitude, there should be a corresponding physical change. If dance therapy brings about a change in the body's behavior, there should be a corresponding change in the mind (Schoop and Michell, cited in Lewis, 1986, p. 46)

. . . the link between physical and mental activity is little understood. The whole field of psychosomatic medicine has only recently been recognised as a valid field of study, and there are many differing opinions about the influence of the mind on the body and vice versa (Lamb, 1965, p. 9).

In first section of this chapter, following a brief discussion of what dance/movement therapy is, the authors describe the goals of therapy. Next, they describe the results of effectiveness and efficacy studies in dance/movement therapy. In third section, the authors describe the differences between movement therapy and strictly verbal interventions.

What Is Dance/Movement Therapy?

Dance/movement therapy involves the use of movement to integrate the mind and body. The process emphasizes the relationship between movement and the primary mother-infant bond, focuses on enhancing the clients' development of world view and self-esteem. ". . . The primacy of body movement in communication and in the development of healthy realistic self and object representations" (Lewis, 1986, p. 142) are central theoretical dispositions promulgated by the use of dance/movement therapy. Dance/movement therapy is the intentional and compassionate use of the elements of movement and dance to promote physical, psychological, and spiritual well being. The process assists clients in contacting with the truth that is inside themselves. However according to Chodorow (1995) ". . . movement at any moment is rarely from a single level of the psyche. Every expressive action reflects the individual mover's attempt to cope dynamically with impulses and images that come from many sources" (p. 112). Different qualities of movement can evoke memories. By experiencing a variety of movements in an authentic way and feeling the movement kinetically, clients begin to get in touch with repressed memories and feelings. Owing to its active engagement and holistic involvement, this intervention can facilitate greater awareness, mastery over body sensations, and corresponding emotions (Thomson, 1997). Ganet-Sigel has suggested that during movement body emotions come out rapidly. As internal feelings are released, clients are able to understand themselves better, to understand why they have certain feelings, and to react in predictable ways. Working through dance/movement therapeutic processes can change the clients' feelings about their body, expand their repertoire of how to view life situations, and alter emotional states.

Historically dance has been used throughout societies and civilizations as a form of communication, to celebrate, to exorcise "bad spirits," or to express basic human emotions (Bartenieff, 1972). Dance and movement awaken the clients' inner lives and can evoke consciousness about their intrapsychic realities (Romero, Hurwitz, & Carranza, 1982). While it is neither purely an intellectual or physical activity, dance/movement becomes an emotional experience that encourages clients to get to know themselves through nonverbal exploration. The potency of dance/movement therapy partly resides in its capacity to evoke communication, promote interaction, and enliven clients in kinesthetic, emotional, spiritual, and cognitive domains. As a holistic modality, it is vitally important in today's medical world and can be used as a complementary therapy to strictly verbal or medicinal approaches to treatment.

Because of its affinity to the arts, dance/movement therapy is grounded in nondiscursive expressions that are more capable of depicting emotional life than discursive language. Common to the modes of art, dance/movement therapy provides a vehicle through which individuals can discover, rediscover, and heal themselves. Emotional wounds may be re-experienced, reshaped, become more understandable, and less potent (Saul, 1988).

There is a parallel development between the mind and body as well as a mutual interdependence between the psyche and the soma (Schur, 1955). The dance/movement therapist can be instrumental in promoting clients' realization that the two are integrally connected. Taking cues from the residue of psychic phenomena left in the body, the therapist identifies movements that help clients recreate homeostasis between the soma and the psyche. Movement is directed towards enhancing an awareness of their physical state en route to an examination of their psychic economy. During the movement process, as clients become aware of the messages that emanate from their soma, perceptions and recognitions of their own and others' bodies increases (Siegel, 1973).

Goals of Dance/Movement Therapy

Dance/movement therapy has been used for the purpose of facilitating client integration. According to Ritter and Low (1996), changes in client functioning may include:

- resocialization and integration within social systems;
- nonverbal creative expression *and emotional catharsis;*
- total self and body awareness and enhanced self-esteem;
- broader movement capabilities and tensions release; and
- enjoyment through relaxation (p. 249).

Lewis (1986) suggests that dance/movement may bring about improvement in the client's: intrapsychic organization, flow of energy, capacity for vitality and relaxation and meaningful social interaction, ability to resolve conflicts, realize potential, meet needs, and maintain an awareness of the present.

The therapeutic process entails creating an awareness, exploration, and the working-through of developmentally related maladaptive experiences so that over time dysfunctional patterns can be replaced by adaptive behaviors. During the process, the therapist observes the client's movement patterns. As the client and therapist begin to establish an alliance, the therapist facilitates the client's awareness and exploration of his/her nonverbal behavior. Movement is used to help bridge conscious and unconscious worlds and bring unconscious material into conscious awareness. The therapist is frequently viewed as a guide into and from the realms of the unconscious and provides ". . . a therapeutic container in which the patient's unconscious can be contacted and embodied" (Lewis, 1986, p. 228). By offering a direct avenue into the unconscious, it is during this process that ". . . unedited material from the unconscious [such as developmentally predisposed psycho-physiologic maladaptions] can be observed, engaged, and re-experienced" (Lewis, 1986, p. 280). In this manner, the therapist ". . . can facilitate an individual's journey and relationship to more universal realms" (Lewis, 1986, p. 283). Stanton (1991) suggested that a person's style of movement may indicate something about his/her personality.

> Theme related and free associational authentic movement, dyadic movement involving the transference/countertransference within the transitional space, and rhythmic or [*theme-based movement*] from the primary process world of the unconscious provides not

only images and verbal reflections, but it can totally engage the person in re-experiencing the developmentally based environments which negatively influenced his natural development (p. 142).

What makes dance/movement therapy so powerful is that the body doesn't lie. Dance/movement therapy helps tap into people's innermost thoughts and feelings as they emerge through the body. While clients can easily be intellectual in verbal therapy, during movement, the body speaks authentically. The veracity of observations is immutable.

Reported Effectiveness and Efficacy of Dance/Movement Therapy

In this section, the authors discuss studies of the effectiveness and efficacy of dance/movement therapy. Seligman (1995) explains how effectiveness and efficacy studies differ. Fundamentally, each type of study asks a different kind of question. The effectiveness study asks what works, how, and why. These studies helps the discerning reader to determine what treatment or intervention works and how clients fare under the actual condition of treatment or intervention. In contrast, the efficacy study seeks to answer the question: Is one intervention more effective than another? The efficacy study can, for example, help the reader determine whether a highly controlled specific treatment or intervention works better than another treatment or control group. A statistical technique called "meta-analysis" is often used to assess the efficacy of psychotherapy. Effect size is employed to assess the magnitude of change or a relationship that is calculated for each intervention study. Effect size is a quantitative method for describing how well the average client who received the same intervention performed relative to the average client who did not receive the intervention. The larger the effect size, the more powerful the intervention. According to Borg and Gall (1989), effect sizes greater than .33 are assumed to large enough to make a worthwhile difference in the outcome.

To better understand the application of meta-analysis, consider the following example. To determine the efficacy of psychotherapy on alcoholism, Schlesinger, Mumford and Glass (1978) conducted a meta-analysis of 20 experiments in which control groups were employed. The dependent variable was to determine the success rate (abstinence or near abstinence). The success rate was 51% for the experimental group, and 31% for the control group. The results suggested that overall psychotherapy was effective. A correlation between the hours of psychotherapy and success rate was reported at .49. Judging the effectiveness of interventions in this way may provide the reader with a better understanding of just how well psychotherapy actually works. Although meta-analysis is not without limitations (See Jackson, 1980; Glass, McGaw, & Smith, 1981; Rosenthal, 1984; Slavin, 1986), this procedure is regarded as the best method for culminating and integrating the results of multiple studies.

How is a meta-analysis conducted?   The process of meta-analysis involves a systematic search of the literature to find articles that meet pre-defined criteria (Lambert & Bergin, 1994). The findings from each study are converted to a common metric, the effect size. Effect size is computed by subtracting the mean score of the control group on the dependent variable from the experimental group mean and dividing by the control group standard deviation. The effect size expresses the difference between group means in standard deviation units. The mean effect size for all of the studies included in a meta-analysis is calculated to estimate the typical effect of the variable under study (Borg & Gall, 1989).

Below the authors describe studies that explore the impact of dance/movement therapy with (a) children, (b) females, (c) substance abusers, (d) psychiatric clients, (e) the elderly, and (f) across cultures, and the implications for collaborating with educators. This section is devoted to helping the reader acquire an understanding to the following questions. What happens to the client who engages in movement? How does the therapist know what the client has experienced? How does the client come to understand what he/she has experienced? The body, with its mode of communication, a language that exceeds the boundaries of verbalizations and conveys kinesthetic, motoric and sensory expressions, may give way to alternate ways of understanding cognitions and symbolic representations. Movement experiences bring to consciousness experiences that were previously nonverbal or preverbal. How does the revelation of previously unexpressed experiences aid the client in a process of self-discovery or healing? As Koren (1994) observed, movement becomes both ". . . a gateway and a medium for the unfolding unity of being" (p. 33). Movement reveals the ". . . inner genuine truth of one's own being channeled through kinesthetic sensation . . ." (Koren, 1994, p. 33) and provides a bridge to understanding the synthesis of the client's lived verbal and non-verbal experiences.

Dance/Movement Therapy and Children

Dance/movement therapy has been reported to be an effective intervention in working with children who suffer from multiple disabilities. Lasseter, Privette, Brown, and Duer (1989) observed that a 12 year old girl with cerebral palsy, mild mental retardation, and emotional problems demonstrated marked motor development improvement, experienced positive feelings about herself, school, and social situations, and began experiencing age appropriate activities with her peers. As a result of dance/movement therapy, changes in motor, an increase of 12 credited months, were measured by the Oseretsky Tests of Motor Proficiency. The Coopersmith Self-Esteem Inventory demonstrated substantial increases in activities measured by the self, social, school, and life subscales. This study indicated that by encouraging relationships between the child and the therapist or other children, dance/movement therapy can be highly effective for children who have problems of self-concept and inhibited interpersonal relations, difficulty expressing personality, and impaired motor development.

Partelli (1995) has emphasized that it is crucial for the dance/movement therapist to listen and observe movement in order to understand the stereotypic and bodily distortions characteristic of children with autism and psychosis. She claimed that the therapist's ability to analyze the child's movement patterns and yet listen with their eyes is similar to a mother's kinesthetic receptiveness and empathy for her baby. As the therapist builds an alliance with the child and they move together rhythmically, he/she can help the child to elaborate and integrate his/her movement and begin to engage the client in an externalized dialogue. Partelli presented two case studies and explained how the process can be used to: (1) shape a facilitating environment suited to the client's needs, (2) create a dialogue that will support integration of movement, images, and emotions, (3) encourage the healthy expression of mental functioning, and (4) support the clients' emergening perception of themselves, others, and the world around them.

Goodill (1987) suggested that dance/movement can be a useful intervention for children who have been abused. Many victims of abuse have unclear and confused boundaries about the personal space of others and their own. They can be overtly intrusive with others and protective and distant about their own space. They may be unreceptive to touch or even recoil from those who reach out to them in a nurturing manner. Verbally approaching an abused child, criticizing, or using of harsh tones may produce a startle effect or cowering. Through dance/movement therapy, the therapist can provide an environment that offers safety, predictability, and interactions that may lead to the desensitization of traumatic incidents and recurrent responses.

Dance/movement can be used to help children who are victims of abuse express unconscious experiences. If the memories that victims of abuse have endured are prior to language development and are pre-verbal, nonverbal or nonverbalizable, they are devoid of cognitive schemata. Dance/movement therapy can also assist these clients in defining and exercising control of their own space and gaining a sense of control over and ownership for their bodies. In the therapeutic environment, abused children are able to learn about nurturing touch, how to determine if a person is safe to be with, and what to do if they sense their safety is in jeopardy. Goodill suggests that clients will need to work through traumatic experiences in stages, commensurate with their tolerance for discomfort and pain and cognitive development, the degree of trauma, and support systems. She cautions, however, that issues related to abuse are likely to re-surface as clients experience physical changes, new relationships, and social demands. Both therapist and client should understand the imperative for working on issues over time at increasingly higher levels of insight and understanding.

Shennum (1987) explored the impact of art and dance/movement therapy on children who were receiving treatment in a residential center. The sample included 42 children ranging in age from 6.7 to 12.8 years, 27 males, and 15 females. Sixty-seven percent of the sample was Caucasian, 19% was Black, 2% were from Hispanic and other ethnic/racial groups. The children in this study had suffered from a variety of behavioral and emotional problems. Abuse and neglect was observed among many of these children. Thirty-three percent had been physically and sexually abused, 12% had been neglected, and 29% were abused and neglected. Results of ANOVA were statistically significant for the children who received treatment on measures of emotional unresponsiveness and behavioral acting-out. Children who received a greater amount of expressive art therapy tended to be less emotionally unresponsive and showed less behavioral acting out than those who received less therapy. While this study did not distinguish what behavioral changes could be attributed specifically to art or dance/movement therapy, the findings highlight the benefits of expressive therapy in a residential milieu.

In a concept paper, Creadick (1985) reported that Feder and Feder (1981) had observed how dance/movement has fostered growth among retardates and individuals with paralysis. Withdrawn individuals were observed to emerge from the shadows of withdrawal and passivity. Retardates began to speak more clearly and those suffering from paralysis began to demonstrate motion in their limbs. Dance/movement therapy as well as other expressive art therapies have been used successfully in the treatment of children who suffer from handicapping conditions. Through these processes, therapists receive qualitative information that helps them understand the physical and psychological growth that children have made.

Dance/Movement for Female Clients

In an anecdotal report of her work with over 40 women who experienced long-term dance/movement therapy over a seven year period, Meyer (1985) described how dance/movement therapy has been used to help women clients explore a wider range of dilemmas. Clients' therapeutic issues were comprised by developing alternatives to dominant/submissive roles in relationships, exploring feelings of helpfulness, passivity, getting in touch with their feelings, feeling their bodies, experiencing freedom from conformity and stereotypical images of women, softening their inner critic, and experiencing a release from socially sanctioned false humility. Meyer (1985) offered insight about its effectiveness. Working with a woman who felt conflicted by a discongruence between her own desires and parental and societal expectations revealed how dance/movement therapy helped to close the gap between external self-image and inner experience. Leventhal & Chang (1991) have suggested that it is the process of "physicalizing inner realities" that permits an integration of experiences into consciousness and acknowledges a fuller experience of selfhood.

> . . . externalizations and physicalization are the mechanisms through which behavior, perception, and insight interface (Leventhal & Chang, 1991, p. 137).

The process of dance/movement has also been used to offer female clients a special place in which they were able to reveal parts of themselves that were typically censored or unacknowledged in other therapeutic settings. However, a woman's comfort or familiarity with movement determines the degree of risk-taking that she can cope with at any given time. Meyer (1985) discovered ". . . that women clients [should] not be pushed to resolve issues before they are ready . . ." (p. 8). Instead she recommended that they be encouraged to ". . . find their own pace and path through any apparent impasse, moving through when the time is ripe" (p. 8). Leventhal and Chang (1991) also suggested that permitting clients to determine their own pace and intensity is crucial to self-control and catalyzing feelings of powerfulness. They suggested that as women worked through conflicts, their observable movements and expressed thought patterns revealed impasses to an enlarged range of conceptual and emotional choices.

A woman's psychological state and perceptions of herself may also influence capacity for self-choice. In work with battered women, Leventhal and Chang (1990) observed that learned helplessness was crucial in women's inability to perceive alternatives for changes. They observed that dance/movement therapy evoked symbolic representations of unconscious and cognitive beliefs and fostered battered women's capacity for choice and independent action. They found that "the creativity and activity inherent to these processes can replace ingrained patterns of immobilization" (Leventhal and Chang, 1991, p. 140), reduce self-blame and alienation, encourage feelings of cohesion, and enhance the clients' capacity to explore pragmatic solutions.

Research has revealed a relationship between field independence and field dependence and psychiatric disorders. According to Reiland (1990), Patients with psychosis and hallucinations, ulcers, asthma, obesity, depression, anorexia, heroin addictions, and character disorders tend towards field dependence. These patients also suffer from a blurring of boundaries, an inability to distinguish between aspects of the environment and self. Psychiatric patients that tend towards field independence include individuals with delusional psychosis, schizoprehenia, paranoia, and obsession-compulsion. Suffering from rigidity of boundaries, these patients often exhibit a marked inability to form close attachments. Alcoholics tend towards field dependence. An inability to distinguish between the effects of alcohol use, perceptions and interactions with others fosters the cycle of denial that often mitigates against recovery. However, dance/movement therapy can help the client re-experience early attachments with the primary caregiver, recapitulate missed opportunities to individuate and develop more accurate body image and an articulated sense of body boundaries.

Dance/movement therapy has been instrumental in helping field dependent clients move towards field independence. In her work with four alcoholic women, Reiland (1990) observed that therapy enabled clients to move towards field independence. Overall the clients demonstrated an ability to distinguish and articulate to feel separate and distinct. These results are preliminary and the author offers cautionary notes. Methodologically, the study suffered from serious limitations (a small sample, a lack of a control group and longitudinally, and an imprecise measure of field independence-dependence). Despite this, Reiland's study highlights the need for future research to help illuminate the role that dance/movement therapy may play in the process of separation-individuation as it relates to cognitive style.

Dance/Movement Therapy and the Substance Abuser

Just as addiction does, dance/movement therapy deals foremost with the body (Perlmutter, 1992). The therapeutic process give clients an opportunity to form a new and different relationship with their bodies and a means to express feelings that often lack words. Although little research has been documented about the effectiveness of dance/movement with this population, Milliken (1990) has suggested that a nonverbal body-oriented approach can be useful in treating the substance abuser's resistance and lack of body awareness and helpful in identifying the underlying issues that may foster addiction. Dance/movement therapy is more aligned with a belief that addiction is caused by ego deficits and internal conflict rather than a biologically determined disease process. Using this intervention, clients can reveal the feelings of insecurity, shame, loss, humiliation, denial, anger, embarrassment, emptiness, alienation, powerfulness, and perversions of sexuality that may have led them to addiction without fear of being judged (Perlmutter, 1992).

Consistent with the ego deficit model, dance/movement therapy has been used to de-differentiate the fused or field-dependent substance abuse client, reduce globalization of a flood of feelings that lead to the experience of unbearable and uncontrollable anxiety, and rebuild a dysfunctional system of defenses. For example, group experiences may be formulated around building the clients': (a) capacity to identify and tolerate feelings, (b) establish trust in self and others, (c) identify losses, and (d) build a repertoire of adaptive coping mechanisms and behavioral responses (Milliken 1990). The act of moving with others in group therapy leads to feelings of cohesion and belongingness and offers a medium to experience and create different type of social interactions.

A meaningful and complete approach to the treatment of alcoholism must consider the interactions between alcohol and social, psychological, and biological functions. Understanding the etiology of ego impairments that foster this illness may also hold crucial information that can be used to guide treatment. Fisher (1990) reported the efficacy of the adjunctive use of dance/movement therapy in treating alcoholics in a 28-day hospital program. She suggested that this approach led to improved self-esteem, exploration of alternative approaches to life circumstances, integration of mind and body, self-acceptance, and spontaneity for patients who were experiencing phases of early recovery.

Dance/Movement Therapy for Psychiatric Clients

Overall there is a dearth of research on the effectiveness of dance/movement with psychiatric populations. However, as the studies reported below suggest, dance/movement may be an effective intervention for this population of clients. Several researchers (Westbrook & McKibben, 1989; Farelly & Joseph, 1991; Heber, 1993; Grodner, Braff, Janowsky, & Clopton, 1982; Romero, Hurwitz, & Carranza, 1983) reported the benefits of dance/movement therapy for clients suffering from Parkinson's disease, major psychiatric disorders, or from an acute crisis. Citing the work of Adler (1974), Kalish (1974), Wise (1981) and Berrol and Katz (1985), Westbrook and McKibben (1989) reported that dance/movement therapy has been effective in the treatment of traumatic brain and spinal cord injury, stroke, multiple sclerosis, autism and sensory loss. Among the changes observed were: increased body and emotional awareness, improved body image and an enlivened sense of physical and emotional well-being. Westbrook and McKibben (1989) observed clients with Parkinson's disease in an exercise group and dance/movement therapy groups. After comparing the movement and mood of clients in each group, they found that the dance/movement therapy group demonstrated improvements in their walking speed and duration of walking time. Subjective improvements in mood were also observed in the dance/movement group. Despite the methodological limitations of the study (inability to account for the bias due to different group leaders, mortality, small sample size, the need for additional measures to assess mood changes), the authors recommended that dance/movement therapy might be a useful adjunctive approach in the treatment of Parkinson's disease.

Crisis intervention services have also used dance/movement therapy. These services are provided to individuals who seek relief from emotionally charged situations. Often times, clients are in need of brief psychotherapy in order to regain control in the face of an overwhelming circumstance. Observing that many clients experience muscular tension, shallow breathing, and postural construction, Farrelly and Joseph (1991) described the benefits of brief intervention of dance/movement therapy on one crisis intervention services client. Movement and breathing exercises were implemented for a client who reported she was "going crazy" and requested medication. Following this intervention, the client demonstrated reduced anxiety, a more relaxed posture and expressed a sense of full relief. The client was later released without medication. Although the researchers did not determine if the effects of treatment were temporal or sustained, the reduction of anxiety, visceral improvements and the patient's sense of satisfactory relief suggest that a salutary outcome was achieved. In another case involving a crisis group, Farrelly and Joseph (1991) observed that when movement was combined with verbalization, clients' ability to focus on the attainment of short-term goals was enhanced. Additionally, clients demonstrated increased interaction, heightened empathy, and an improved ability to experience togetherness.

Dance/movement has been used to help many psychiatric clients overcome isolation, alienation, or withdrawal and to mobilize the under-active or depressed (Heber, 1993). This study was designed to measure the impact of dance/movement therapy on clients who suffered from anxiety, tension, depression and low self-esteem. Followed through case study analyses and intellectualized responses (N=204), clients revealed that they experienced a reduction in tension and apprehension. They also exhibited dramatic changes in self-attitudes and increased communication with peers. Heber concluded that dance/movement therapy helped clients integrate emotional, cognitive and spiritual dimensions. Additionally, some clients who were unable to move actively because they were taking high doses of medication reported positive feelings towards the use of dance/movement. To date, the author has recorded the results for more 350 participant-clients.

Grodner, Braff, Janowsky, and Clopton (1982) designed a study to measure the effects of art and movement on 3 groups of 15 participants, 12 with major psychiatric disorders (psychosis or depression) and 3 staff members. Participants were assigned to either directed or nondirected art/movement therapy group, or no treatment group. The results suggested that the combined art/movement therapy group temporarily improves mood and social interactions. The design of the study prohibited the researchers from determining whether changes were the result of one or both therapies, the therapy itself or the use of directed activity. The final results may have been biased since participants who didn't complete their ratings scales were not included in the final sample. The effect of therapist on the groups was also not assessed. Moreover, it was difficult to separate the degree to which improvements were caused by movement, art or the use of psychotropic drugs, although the authors claimed that improvement due to the therapy was at least equal to those caused by the drugs.

Most schizophrenics suffer from an impaired ability to communicate their intrapsyhic reality and function adaptively in interpersonal relationships. However, despite these limitations, Romero, Hurwitz, and Carranza (1982) have observed that schizophrenics can communicate through dance/movement therapy. In a theoretical paper based on work with this clinical population, the researchers concluded that this therapy can be a useful adjunct in the treatment of acute and chronic schizophrenia. Claiming that dance/movement therapy has many benefits, they reported that clients ". . . begin to perceive that they have an image to present to themselves . . ." (p. 88) and others, believe the space they occupy is important, demonstrate increasingly flexible and more complex movement, and improved body image, self-esteem, and social interactions. They highlighted the importance of establishing clear boundaries and delineating the therapist-patients' roles during group work.

Dance/Movement Therapy and the Elderly

There have been few studies regarding the effectiveness of dance/ movement therapy with the elderly. In 1978, Sandel implemented a movement program for geriatric patients in a convalescent home. The purposes of the program was to promote socialization and increase patients' sensory stimulation with non-rigorous movement. Low-intensity movement has been reported to improve the elasticity of muscles and joints and relieve stress (Samberg, 1988). In fact, even as early as 1925, Schilder observed that: "Movement is a great uniting factor between the different parts of one's own body" (p .112).

Initially, Sandel formed a group of eight men and women who ranged in age from 77 to 91. After establishing clear boundaries and explaining that the group was only for patient interaction, group cohesion was achieved by the eighth session. A second and more functional group was convened later. This group was comprised of seven men and women who ranged in age from 73 to 98. After about two months, with a core of six members, this group achieved considerable stability.

The groups permitted patients to an opportunity to share feelings and memories, encouraged physical contact, and verbalization. Group actions such as giving and taking became important therapeutic strategies (Lindner, 1982). As a result of their movement experiences, patients' spontaneous expressions of feelings, assertive behaviors, conversation before and after sessions as well as interactions during sessions increased. Group members began to reaffirm the emotional interactions that the physical relationship of the movement stimulated (Lindner, 1982) and improve social interactions (Samberg, 1988). An increase in patient stamina and a greater variety of movement was observed. Staff reported changes in patients' behaviors in large groups: increased socialization and greater responsiveness to music. A greater willingness to do exercises or creative movement activities at other recreational events was also observed. Issues that emerge during group may provide opportunities for diagnosis and constructive change by either the therapist or in conjunction with other professionals.

Lindner (1982) suggested that dance/movement therapy can improve the elderly's sense of well-being and help them deal with the psychosocial stress associated with the process of aging and institutionalization. This therapy also becomes a demonstration even to infirm and aged adults that their physical bodies need not be a burden to them but can be a source of pleasure (Samberg, 1988). Also, for patients who suffer from aphasia and other speech disorders, an alternative means of communication can be provided. This approach has also been instrumental in evoking brief cognitive reorganization among confused patients. Unique to the social, nonverbal playful, and physically concrete context that dance/movement provides, movement holds promise for helping older adults experience a greater sense of unity, self-esteem, communication, and physical well-being. Dance/movement therapy along with other expressive therapies, allows the elderly to reach beyond inertia and apathy to experience an array of emotions that later may give way to heightened cognition and finally interaction with the patient's external world (Saul, 1988).

Dance/Movement Therapy Across Cultures

Dance/movement therapy can play a significant role in healing individuals across diverse cultures. Recently, it was introduced to Asians. During Ganet-Sigel's trip to China, Linda Cao observed the impact that dance/movement therapy workshops had upon participants (Ganet-Sigel, 1994). Cao offered several examples.

> . . . "I didn't know how I should move and what I should do," said a student in the first workshop. Jane suggests his problem may be that he couldn't make choices for himself without advice or direction. In the second workshop, when Jane suggested participants say their own name to themselves quietly as they walked through the room, another student shared his feelings, saying, "I am used to introduce myself to other people or tell them who I am on the phone very easily, but I never tell myself who I am. I felt so strange saying my own name to myself" (p .71).
>
> Some people may think that since China has a history of Tai Chi and Martial Arts movements, they should accept Dance/Movement Therapy easily. From the point of body/mind coordination, it is true, but from the point of individual psychotherapy, it may become a restriction or obstacle to the Chinese. All those traditional movements made the Chinese good at moving in the same direction and same routines, but not in moving in an individual way. Chinese focus on holding the body in balance, but have difficulty moving freely. For this reason Dance/Movement Therapy is especially helpful for the Chinese. I can't forget how a young girl several times put herself into Jane's arms and hugged Jane tightly, even though she didn't know her. The child's body was telling us she needed emotional nurturing so much. . . . (p. 72).

Dance/movement therapy has also been cited as an important intervention for working with Native Americans who suffer from mental illness (Dufrene & Coleman, 1994). Native Americans view dance as indistinct from both worship and healing. However, because they combine various arts into healing and spiritual ceremonies, dance/movement therapy, as well as other forms of expressive therapy offer clients a medium in which to: (a) return to their origins, (b) confront and manipulate evil, (c) experience death and rebirth, and (d) restore unity (p. 146). Inherent to the function of dance/movement therapy is the commonality it shares with indigenous healing. The latter is grounded in mythology that views art, healing, and religion as indistinct. Within this framework, the individual can experience a symbolic world and feel familiar, safe, and comfortable. In a similar manner, dance/movement therapy allows clients to experience safety and security, and provides a medium to symbolically relive, reveal, and reconstruct past traumas and experiences that have compromised their functional capacities.

Therapeutic interventions must be responsive to both client malady and the context in which services are delivered. In this realm, viewing the applicability of treatment interventions in context of a cultural frame seems imperative. There is an emergent awareness that physical and emotional health are not limited to the sphere of technological interventions or Eurocentric counseling techniques. However, the Western emphasis on overcoming forces, rather than seeking to understand our own inner responses, mitigates against the use of dance/movement. Many factors in our culture have encouraged divisiveness, including divisions based on gender, race, professional hierarchies, power, and economic status (Canner, 1992). In this light the tension between paradigms of treatment becomes more evident. In the medical model, emphases is placed on diagnosis and cure. However, in the more non-discursive, expressive therapies, the emphasis is on understanding and empowering the individual to heal himself/herself. The interactive nature of physical and mental health highlight the need for providing culturally responsive services to the clients. Dance/movement therapy encourages clients to experience their own creativity and intensifies self-awareness. In treatment of Native Americans, dance/movement therapy may play a vital role in helping clients re-build self-esteem, a sense of belonging, and cultural pride.

Dance/Movement Therapy and Implications for Collaboration with Educators

Dance/movement therapists can play a vital role in the diagnosis and treatment of school-aged children. Diagnostically, therapists could assist educators in the identification of students' sensory and perceptual-motor problems. Therapeutically, they could foster students' emotional development and adaptive interactions, reinforce positive self-image, promote self-awareness, and provide a medium for emotional and creative expression (Canner, 1992).

Rauskin (1990) suggested that dance/movement therapy can be useful in special education settings. This intervention can support and enhance the acquisition of educational skills and social, emotional, and behavioral goals detailed in students' individualized educational plans. Moreover, dance/movement can help to ameliorate deficiencies that impede learning. She pointed out that movement can be used to address reading problems such as visual discrimination, memory, and directionality. While advocating for a particular model of group therapy with children with emotional disturbance, she stresses that group processes provide children with tools fundamental to learning how to solve problems, be creative, make decisions, and master other basic cognitive skills.

With the federal legislation of P. L. 94–142, and the push for full-service schools, dance/movement therapists may find a greater welcoming in schools. Many contemporary educators have acknowledged the value of working alongside with non-instructional personnel to diagnose students' maladies, develop appropriate individualized educational plans, and to maximize students' learning experiences. The collaboration between educators and mental health workers is becoming viewed as an important enterprise in fostering children's health and in the prevention of mental illness.

Summary of Effectiveness and Efficacy Studies in Dance/Movement Therapy

Overall there is a dearth of rigorous research in the field and very few controlled studies that evaluate its effectiveness (Payne, 1988; Ritter & Low, 1996). Many of the studies that the authors cited are theoretical, descriptive, or case study approaches; others are studies of effectiveness. Although many studies reported in the literature suffer serious methodological limitations, the evidence revealed provides a compelling case that dance/movement therapy is an effective therapeutic intervention for bringing about the restoration of health. Ritter and Low (1996) have suggested that other important studies may have remained unpublished because the findings lacked statistical significance. In their meta-analysis of 23 studies, the authors reported that dance/movement therapy has had a positive impact for clients who suffer from anxiety and that adults and adolescents benefit more than children. However they cautioned that additional research is needed. They reported that overall research suffers from serious methodological problems and that there were few well-designed experiments that have assessed the effectiveness of dance/movement therapy. While recognizing the benefits of this intervention for adults and adolescents, they suggested that further in-depth research is needed to substantiate qualitative findings.

Differences Between Dance/Movement and Strictly Verbal Interventions

Early approaches to verbal psychotherapy failed to integrate an emphasis on the mind-body connection to the degree that this connection has been explored and confirmed during the past fifty years. As early as the 1940's and 1950's, modern dancers used the dance medium to develop an understanding of the relationship between the mind and the body. Since movement is one of the initial human experiences, it offers a unique medium to facilitate memories stored during pre-verbal communication and to bring about alternative modes of communication. Dance/movement therapy among other expressive arts therapies, places a value on non-verbal communication. The use of movement has been effective in treating clients who were unreachable verbally or in cases where their psychiatric issues were related to their physical body, directly or indirectly.

Long before infants have the capacity to verbalize their physical and emotion needs, they are completely dependent upon their primary caregiver for nurturance, sustenance, and appropriate responses to address their most basic needs. The caregiver must carefully read their body language in order to understand their cries, smiles, coos, or despair. Attunement and empathic responses to the infant are major functions of the primary caregiver. However, oftentimes, the healthy and dysfunctional messages children receive during childhood become ingested viscerally. As the emergening child begins to individuate and develop his/her own personality, viscerally stored feelings and memories are unconsciously broadcast in his/her movement patterns. When messages or experiences are unhealthy or traumatic, the quality of visceral communication may become more extreme and dysfunctional, affecting both the child's perception of experiences or impairing his/her ability to filter out, rather than merge with others' maladaptive behaviors.

Dance/movement therapy allows clients to return to their roots and relive experiences that occurred during childhood and the preverbal developmental phase. Although the extent to which clients may re-experience events may be affected by their intellectual capacity and the psyche's capacity to permit relevations, the potential to heal deeply repressed somatic memories or preverbal traumas is significant. During the dance/movement process, clients often enter a transcendental state, in which their creative potential supersedes the cognitive skills. Dance/movement therapy offers a dynamic and distinctive approach to helping clients reveal, release, and reconstruct as their intrapsychic pain moves to a conscious level of awareness. Therapeutically, clients may benefit from dance/movement therapy, since the revelation of issues that gave rise to dysfunction shifts the locus of control for healing squarely upon the clients,' rather than the therapists' shoulders. While the authors unequivocally advocate for the use of dance/movement therapy as an alternative approach to treating psychiatric disorders, neurosis, emotional and behavioral disturbance, they also suggest that whether dance/movement therapy is used as the primary or adjunctive mode of treatment is best left to the discretion of therapists overseeing clients' care. However, they stress that dance/movement therapy is a viable and efficacious modality that should be seriously considered.

Claiming the therapeutic efficacy of dance/movement therapy and other creative arts therapies in their own right, Gibson (1980) observed that it evokes response more immediately than more traditional verbal therapy. He also observed the cultural and educational value of this intervention.

> The creative arts therapies are uniquely suited to meet certain needs of the underserved — the children and adolescents, ethnic minorities, the chronically ill. Many patients in these underserved groups are not readily accessible to verbal therapies . . . Language barriers created by ethnic and socioeconomic differences are tran-

scended by the nonverbal communication of the creative arts. Children and adolescents often can express themselves and relate only through the shared artistic experience (p. 6).

Lewis (1996) has suggested that through verbal psychotherapy clients may gain an intellectual understanding of their feelings. However, often very little healing has occurred, because the etiology of the primary issues remains deep inside, untouched, unchanged. Philosophically, dance/movement therapy is grounded in the belief that the body and mind work in ongoing reciprocal interactions. What affects the mind affects the body. What affects the body, affects the mind. Until clients have acquired a visceral understanding, it is unlikely that therapeutic intervention will evoke enduring change. Change occurs when clients have integrated intellectual awareness with somatic understanding.

Based upon the conviction that unconscious material resides in the body, the embodied process inherent to movement can permit clients to fully experience, own, and transform the emotions that have fostered maladaptive functioning. Clients aren't likely to find a rapid remedy in this modality. As one client expressed, to achieve healing, clients must be willing to sustain the intense feelings that may accompany the revelation of memories repressed in the soma.

> I think it's very important that, that a client needs to stay with it. Too many times I've seen people leave group or run away, because an issue might have touched some points that were too rough, or too painful, or they just weren't ready to deal with yet. I think it's very important to give the process time and to be patient with it, to stick with it so that you can get the full benefits from it. A few sessions isn't going to do it. A lot of people think they can like go to verbal therapy and in a few sessions be cured — but that's not healing. No effective change can occur in a "quick fix."

While movement can help clients address early childhood memories, it is unlikely that habitual movements or dysfunctional patterns are going to lie down and die. This means that clients have to work on building strengths and new adaptations and neutralizing the defensive structures. Once adaptive behaviors have been internalized enough they will overpower the dysfunctional behaviors which will be able to die a quiet and conscious death (Lewis, 1986).

Naturally there can be significant benefits to clients using a combined approach of verbal and movement therapy. As one former client, now a colleague, observed:

> I think that all of those modalities are very good. [However], in any kind of movement modality it is impossible to hide behind words. And if you work with a really, really competent gifted practitioner, there's a certain natural distinction or eye that the [dance/movement therapist] has that cannot be compared to any kind of verbal modality where the two people are kind of sitting and facing each other and there's no movement other than verbal. Although a psy-

chologist, a social worker, or psychiatrist may be well trained in what we're calling "body language" these days, it's not the same as getting — what I call "getting into the trenches." Dance/movement therapists do actually get in with the patient or client and move with them so that the experience is shared, which makes it a lot less threatening. And it also validates the client's feelings by saying: "I will move with you, and share in your process and journey."

Dance/movement therapy offers a mechanism to enlarge the verbal psychotherapist's perspective of the client's level of functioning. Logistically, verbal and movement therapy could be used in a complementary fashion since the therapeutic dance/movement therapy session includes a verbal component in which clients are invited to discuss and work through the experiences they had during the process of movement.

Some psychotherapeutic researchers have asked: Do clients benefit by getting in touch with their feelings? While this question is not easily answered, some researchers have raised questions about the sustainability of psychotherapy. Allen (1980) claimed that while it has been assumed that focus on affect has a lasting impact, little is known about the specific means for bringing about an enhanced capacity for affect experience. In contrast the movement process really cuts through facades and allows clients to look at themselves and permits someone else to share as a witness. Movement permits observation without the mask of verbiage and invites a therapist to offer his/her assessment and say "Here's what it looks like you're doing or what you're going through." The therapist's interpretation may catalyze clients' awareness, insight, or surprise, such as indicated in the feelings expressed by: "I never thought about that. You're right." The movement process can then give way to a process of unfolding, exploration, analysis, and metamorphosis.

The process puts clients in a place that is almost a trancelike state. This is a place where we go unconsciously, where the actual healing process happens. One of the individuals that was interviewed, a practicing dance/movement therapist, suggested that there are three levels of awareness that pertain to client expression and movement. Levels one and two relate to the client. Level three results from client-therapist interaction. Level one is comprised by the client's description of how he/she perceives him/herself. Level two is characterized by the interaction between the client's unconscious and his/her core body movement. For example, level two could be described as consisting of a particular individual, with his/her unconscious and all of his/her unconscious experiences, feelings, and perceptions. Level three requires the therapist to synthesize his/her observations and interpretations simultaneously to read what it is that they're seeing and to interpret what it is that they're seeing. Therapists are not interpreting on a conscious plane either, because what they're doing is viscerally feeling what they're seeing, experiencing, and feeling. Therapists will articulate their physical and visceral experiences and share their impressions with the clients. Another practicing dance/movement therapist offered additional insight about the process.

Movement is used to put someone into a creative frame of mind. Sometimes people are not aware when they are in a creative frame of mind. Movement is facilitated by the dance/movement therapist to help someone get into a flow. Flow is a different type of consciousness or mentality. The process of flow is different for each person, the nature of flow is developmental. The quality of flow tends to be intrinsic to each person even though each person can develop ways of tapping into it. From there the client experiences a deeper and wider perspective of what is going on with him or her.

Since a lot of people don't know how to get at it or identify it in themselves, how can this process be influenced by the therapist and his/her use of movement techniques? To help clarify the nature of this relationship, a practicing dance/movement therapist stated that:

It is really up to clients and whether they are willing to explore and expand their own creativity. Remember that therapeutic interventions are very client-focused. The therapist builds on what the client presents. Therapy is process-oriented. It depends on the client's ability and/or willingness to become one with the process, to experiment, take risks and to become involved in the movement or theme. This in turn helps the dance/movement therapist read and gather more information in which to present other facilitating kinds of experiences. For example, the dance/movement therapist will try to select a theme for movement that relates to what she sees in people's bodies during the warm-up exercise.

While at times a specific theme doesn't relate to a specific client, as the person begins to move it along with other group members, the universality of the thematic movement takes over. Individuals can still benefit from the theme even though it may not be very powerful for them, because it may not be exactly what they were dealing with in their body. This particular movement process may open doors to issues that clients didn't even know they were dealing with. For example, the therapist might request that clients work in dyads and triads during group therapy. Although under other circumstances clients might not choose to interact with these individuals outside the therapeutic environment, the work they do during therapy can be helpful in other social interactions such as the workplace. Moving with others also helps develop frustration tolerance.

The body expresses what is in unconsciousness. Over time, the client's awareness and ability to listen to his/her consciousness heightens while tolerance for unconscious material increases. the client's adeptness at dipping into the unconscious leads to increased use of body and muscle expression which leads to releasing. Expression and awareness lead to releasing while putting form to stream of consciousness. The client's skill at taking apart the meaning of movement develops. The client gives voice to what the movement triggered (a memory or association).

The therapist will recognize that clients don't always talk directly about the movement, even though in their discussions after the movement portion of the session, they talk about both their movements and feelings. Though clients may not refer specifically to the movement that occurred in the therapy session, what they may talk about is triggered by the movement or the theme used to guide the movement session even though a person may not talk about how a foot was lifted or an arm was raised. Clients will give voice to what was triggered by the movement, such as a past memory, a different type of association. While their verbiage might seem unrelated to the movement, it is intimately related to the movement.

> A person may come into a session upset about something and then they may get into movement. Well as they get into the techniques, they begin to explore that upsetness in a different way, so there is another level of awareness that begins to develop as a result of putting movement to what is this upsetness about. Part of synthesizing that awareness is the talking afterwards. Afterwards you are coming at it from a different angle, a slightly different level of awareness from what you had before you came to the session.

Summary

Through early socialization individuals learn how to be indirect rather than say things clearly. An emphasis is often placed on being inauthentic and concealing feelings. In dance/movement therapy it is impossible for the client to be inauthentic because the body tells all; it is harder to deny what you just did. During therapy, the client's need to explore his/her own feelings and explore the feelings that underlie the movement become very powerful. The process of dance/movement therapy is a mirror of the development of an infant. Every client has his/her own pace, rate, and speed and depth and what he/she can tolerate. Not every client can do the same kind of work. Not every client can be responded to in the same way. Some people cannot take a lot of confrontation, while others cannot. The process of dance/movement therapy is extremely powerful because it puts people in touch with their true, natural selves. One practicing dance/movement therapist described the process as follows:

> Metaphorically . . . it's like there's a river that is all covered with ice. The ice is all the trauma, the defenses and *other maladaptive coping mechanisms.* Clients can either chip away the ice, or go right to the river, and let the river break it up. I think that dance/movement therapy is going to the river. It's going to the river of life, the river of movement and the river of self. When you help people touch that, the healing comes from the inside out.

This quotation exemplifies Jane Ganet-Sigel's core philosophy that dance/movement therapy helps clients release, reveal, and reconstruct.

Conclusions

The therapist can help in conveying experience and knowledge to others by recording case studies, and should not feel guilty about avoiding research (North, 1995, p. 10).

Research constitutes an integral component of exemplary teaching and is an important tool for articulating new knowledge and informing others.

Linda S. Behar-Horenstein, 1999

The research concerning the efficacy of dance/movement therapy has been largely anecdotal, descriptive, or case study in format (Payne, 1988; Ritter & Low, 1996). While much of the research offers compelling insight and leads the reader to believe that dance/movement therapy may be highly effective and efficacious in bringing about sustained healing, conducting a larger body of systematic and methodologically rigorous studies may permit the larger therapeutic community to fully appreciate the validity of this unique modality.

Research and case material in this textbook suggest that movement may evoke a physiological changes that occur concomitantly or alongside with the psychological and behavioral changes that clients experience and exhibit. It seems incumbent that dance/movement therapists view this invitation to share their work as a crucial step in having this field accepted into the range of therapeutic interventions as a partner rather than a fledgling step-child. The benefits of enlarging the scope of research is based on the following beliefs. Many of the cases and vignettes in this textbook highlight the credibility and effectiveness of dance/movement therapy. However, reports in this text represent only a subset of many other undocumented cases. By creating a compendium of methodologically rigorous studies and compiling quantitative and qualitative databases, the efficacy of this therapeutic approach can be made available to others. Moreover, providing comprehensive evidence can serve to demonstrate what numerous authors have already suggested. Secondly, dance/movement therapy has struggled to be accepted as a legitimate form of psychotherapy. Part of the debate stems from a lack of systematic research. However, another problem lies in debates over the cause and effect of emotions and body movement (Rossberg-Gempton and Poole, 1992). They noted that dance/movement therapy ". . . is considered to be an ideal opportunity for the patient to gain a kinesthetic awareness, and maintain a sense of control over movement patterns and the accompanying feelings" (p. 45). Dance/movement therapy, unlike verbal psychotherapy, utilizes a bi-directional approach. A combination of a kinesthetic/emotional/verbal seems more aligned with the socialization norms of our society than solely a preference for intellectual/verbal. Thirdly, if systematic and scientific research studies focused on analysis of muscular movement and affect are conducted, then the field of dance/movement is likely to gain wider acceptance alongside other therapeutic modalities. Adding experimentation to the current observational case study approach will help nullify the controversy surrounding the study of body movement and affect.

Clearly there is a predominance of positivistic, linear, reductionistic methodology in the psychiatric community. However, many of the studies documented in this textbook also used clinical data as well as reports of client experiences. There is ample justification to support the use of the positivistic (quantitative) and postpositivisitic (qualitative) paradigms for research aimed at documenting the effectiveness and efficacy of this approach. There are several ways to enhance the quality of research in dance/movement therapy. The suggestions provided below, while not an exhaustive list, may help to make research findings more accessible to the global therapeutic community.

1. Conduct studies that focus on the determining the efficacy of dance/movement therapy. Follow clients longitudinally to track the sustainability of their progress. Use pre- and post-treatment scales to measure mood or movement changes. If published scales or tests are unavailable, the use of researcher-constructed instruments that have evidence of construct or content validity, as well as reliability measures, may also be suitable to obtain quantitative measures. Compare pre- and post-treatment changes by a variety of variables including: the client's diagnosis, the theoretical approach, the specific dance/therapeutic techniques used and observed, the duration of treatment. Client self-reports of their experiences and changes may also be used to triangulate the findings.

2. Establish the common knowledge base of practices that students are expected to learn and demonstrate during their professional program of study and practice in the field. Quantifying the congruence between the actual behaviors observed in clinic and private practice and those practices taught in the graduate program courses or read in course-related textbooks may help to codify the knowledge base.

3. Study the professional issues that are common to dance/movement therapists professionals at various stages of their career-novice, advanced beginner, and expert and develop a series of recommendations for inservice training that is responsive to the issues related to practitioners at their various experiential levels.

4. Conduct studies that focus on determining the efficacy of dance/ movement therapy according to the therapist's level of expertise.

5. Conduct studies that focus on the determining the efficacy of dance/movement therapy as it relates to the context of the therapeutic setting. Is treatment differentially effective depending upon whether it is conducted in a hospital, residential, convalescent, private, or day-care setting? How does the politics of an institution impact the work that therapists do?

6. In recognition of the preliminary work on the relationship between cognitive styles (field independence and field dependence) and the effects of dance/movement therapy, the following questions could be explored. Do specific treatment approaches for field independent and field dependent clients lead to differential outcomes? Is there a difference between cognitive styles and women and men's responses to dance/movement therapy? Is there a relationship between the client's cognitive style and the effectiveness of dance/movement therapy?

7. Conduct studies to compare the therapist's and client's perceptions about the dance/movement therapy. This would help to bring about a better understanding of the differences between the therapist's and the client's experiences (Payne, 1988).

8. Explore the amount of verbalization that takes place among different therapists who work with similar client populations. Determine the amount of verbalizations between the therapist and client. Determine if vocalizations are an expression of intrapsychic pain or a defense against the therapeutic process. Describe whether the verbalization takes place during the beginning, middle, or end of the movement portion of the session. Determine if there is a relationship between verbalization and the client population, attitudes, values, level of anxiety, development, intelligence, disorder, personality type, or cognitive style (Payne, 1988).

9. Conduct studies that adhere to systematic methods of data analysis. Studies should include random assignment of participants to treatment and control groups, the use of validated measurement instruments, and the use of multivariate statistics to avoid Type I errors (Ritter and Low, 1996).

10. Explore the degree to which group versus individual therapy results in changes in the clients' behaviors (Ritter and Low, 1996).

11. Explore the relationship between the therapists' techniques, adaptations for specific pathologies, and changes in clients' behaviors.

12. When randomization is not possible or when there is an insufficient number of participants, consider the use of qualitative and descriptive techniques to triangulate the findings, while controlling for threats to external and internal validity.

13. Consider using meta-analytic techniques to summarize a collection of findings across related studies.

References

Adler, J. (1974). The study of an autistic child. *ADTA Combined Proceedings from the 3rd and 4th Annual Conference* (pp. 43–48). Columbia, MD: American Dance Therapy Association.

Allen J. (1980). Adaptive functions of affect and their implications for therapy. *The Psychoanalytic Review, 67* (2), 217–220.

American Dance/Movement Therapy Association. (1986). *ATDA manual.* Columbia, MD: American Dance/Movement Therapy Association.

Balint, M. (1968). *The basic fault.* New York and London: Tavistock/Routledge, 1989.

Bartenieff, I. (1972). Dance therapy: A new profession or a rediscovery of an ancient role of the dance? *Dance scope, 7,* 6–18.

Baumann, E. H. (1976). A day treatment program for severely disturbed young children. *Hospital and community psychiatry, 27*(3), 174–179.

Behar-Horenstein, L. S. (1999). Narrative research: Understanding teaching, and teacher thinking. In A. C. Ornstein & L. S. Behar-Horenstein (Eds.). *Contemporary issues in curriculum.* (pp. 90–102). Needham Heights, MA: Allyn & Bacon.

Behar-Horenstein, L. S. (1994). What's worth knowing for teachers? *Educational Horizons, 73*(1), 37–46.

Berelowitz, M. & Tarnopolsky, A. (1993). The validity of borderline personality disorder. In P. Tyrer and G. Stein, *Personality Disorder Reviewed.* (pp. 90–112). London: The Royal College of Psychiatrists.

Berrol, C. & Katz, S. (1985). Dance/movement therapy in the rehabilitation of individuals surviving severe head injuries. *American Journal of Dance Therapy, 8,* 46–66.

Blanck, G. & Blanck, R. (1994). *Ego psychology: Theory and practice.* New York: Columbia University Press.

Blume, E. (1990). *Secret survivors: Uncovering incest and its aftereffects in women.* New York: John Wiley & Sons.

Boerckel, D. & Barnes, C. (1991). *Defeating the banking concept of education: An application of Paulo Freire's methodologies.* Paper presented at the Annual Meeting of the College English Association. San Antonio, TX April 18–20, 1991. Washington, DC: (ERIC Document Reproduction Service No. ED340 017)

Bohlin, R. M., Milheim, W. D., & Viechnicki, K. J. (1993–1994). The development of a model for the design for motivational adult instruction in higher education. *Journal of Educational Technology Systems, 22*(1), 3–17.

Borg, W. R. & Gall, M. D. (1989). *Educational research: An introduction.* Fifth Edition. New York: Longman.

Brown, G. R. & Anderson, B. (1991). Psychiatric morbidity in adult inpatients with childhood histories of sexual and physical abuse. *American Journal of Psychiatry, 148*, 55–61.

Bruch, H. (1978). *The golden cage: The enigma of anorexia nervosa.* Cambridge, MA: Harvard University Press.

Bryne, C. P., Velamoor, V. R., Cernovsky, Z. Z., et al. (1990). A comparison of borderline and schizophrenic patients for childhood lifetime events and parent-child relationships. *Canadian Journal of Psychiatry, 35,* 590–595.

Canner, N. G. (1992). At home on earth. *American Journal of Dance Therapy, 14*(2), 125–131.

Chace, M. (1953). Dance as an adjunctive therapy with hospitalized patients. *Bulletin of Menniger Clinic, 17,* 219–255.

Chaiklin, H., (Ed.). (1975). *Marian Chace: Her papers.* Columbia, MD: American Dance Therapy Association.

Chaiklin, S. (1984). *Dance/movement therapy.* NY: Bain Books.

Cheung, K. C. (1994). *Assessing the quality of learning in higher education: Methods, models and perspectives.* Washington, DC: (ERIC Document Reproduction Service No. ED 381 088)

Chodorow, J. (1995). Body, psyche, and emotions. *American Journal of Dance Therapy, 17*(2), 97–114.

Creadick, T. A. (1985). The role of the expressive arts in therapy. *Journal of Reading, Writing, and Learning Disabilities, 1*(3), 55–60.

Dufrene, P. M. & Coleman, V. D. (1994). Art and healing for Native American Indians. *Journal of Multicultural Counseling and Development, 22*(3), 145–152.

Dunn, R. (1990a). Rita Dunn answers questions on learning styles. *Educational Leadership, 48*(2) 15–19.

Dunn, R. (1990b). Understanding the Dunn and Dunn learning styles model and the need for individual diagnosis and prescription. *Journal of Reading, Writing, and Learning Disabilities, 6*(3), 223–247.

Dunn, R. (1996). *How to implement and supervise a learning style program.* Washington, DC: (ERIC Document Reproduction Service No. ED 395 367)

Dunn, R., Beaudry, J. S., & Klavas, A. (1989). Survey of research on learning styles. *Educational Leadership, 46*(6), 50–58.

Dunn, R., Dunn, K., & Price, G. E. (1989). *Learning styles inventory.* (Available from Price Systems, Box 1818, Lawrence, KS 66044.)

Eisner, E. (1995). Preparing teachers for schools of the 21st century. In Behar-Horenstein, L. S. (Ed). *Peabody Journal of education, 70* (3), pp. 99–111.

Erickson, E. H. (1950). *Childhood and Society.* New York: Norton.

Espenak, L. (1981). *Dance/movement therapy: Theory and practice.* Springfield, IL: Thomas.

Even, M. J. (1982). Adapting cognitive style theory in practice. *Lifelong learning: The adult years.* January, 14–27.

Farrelly, J. & Joseph, A. (1991). Expressive therapies in a crisis intervention service. *The Arts in Psychotherapy, 18,* 131–137.

Feder, E. & Feder, B. (1985). *The expressive arts therapies.* Englewood Cliffs, NJ: Prentice-Hall, Inc.

Fisher, B. (1990). Dance/movement therapy: Its use in a 28-day substance abuse program. *The Arts in Psychotherapy, 17,* 325–331.

Freed, A. O. (1984). Differentiating between borderline and narcissistic personalities. *Social casework: The journal of contemporary social work.* September, 395–404.

Ganet-Sigel, J. (1986). *What is dance/movement therapy?* Unpublished manuscript.

Ganet-Sigel, J. (1994). Dance/Movement Therapy in China. *American Journal of Dance Therapy, 16*(1), 69–72.

Gibson, R. W. (1980). The creative arts therapies: An Overview. *National Association of Private Practice Hospitals, 11*(2), 4–6.

Glaser, B. G. & Strauss, A. L. (1967). *The discovery of grounded theory: Strategies for qualitative research.* Chicago: Aldine.

Glass, G. V., McGaw, B., & Smith, M. L. (1981). *Meta-analysis in social research.* Beverly Hills, CA: Sage.

Goodill, S. (1987). Dance/movement therapy with abused children. *The Arts in Psychotherapy, 14,* 59–68.

Greene, M. (1999). Art and imagination: Overcoming a desperate stasis. In A. C. Ornstein & L. S. Behar-Horenstein, (Eds.). *Contemporary issues in curriculum.* (pp. 45–51). Needham Heights, MA: Allyn & Bacon.

Grodner, S., Braff, D., Janowsky, D., & Clopton, P. (1982). Efficacy of art/movement therapy in elevating mood. *The Arts in Psychotherapy 9,* 217–225.

Hall, C. S. & Lindzey, G. (1998). *Theories of Personality.* Fourth Edition. New York: Wiley and Sons, Inc.

Heber, L. (1993). Dance movement: A therapeutic program for psychiatric clients. *Perspectives in psychiatric care, 29*(2), 22–29.

Herman, J. L. Perry, J. C., & Van Der Kolk, B. A. (1988). Childhood traumas in borderline personality disorder. *American Journal of Psychiatry, 146,* 490–495.

Ignham, J. (1989). *An experimental investigation of the relationships among learning style perceptual preference, instructional strategies, training, achievement, and attitudes of corporate employees.* Unpublished doctoral dissertation. St. John's University, New York.

Jackson, G. B. (1980). Methods for integrative reviews. *Review of Educational Research, 50,* 438–460.

Jackson, L. Barnett, B. Caffarella, R. Lee, P., & Macisaac, D. (Eds.). (1992). *Applying experiential learning in college teaching and assessment: A process model.* Washington, DC: (ERIC Document Reproduction Service No. ED 365 634)

James, W., Mandler, G., & Johnson-Laird, P. N. (1990). The psychology of consciousness. In Pickering, J., & Skinner, M. *From sentience to symbols: Readings on consciousness.* Toronto, Buffalo: University of Toronto Press.

Joughin, G. (1992). Cognitive style and adult learning principles. *International Journal of Lifelong Learning, 11* (1), 3–14.

Joyce, B. R., & Calhoun, E. (1996) *Creating learning experiences: The role of instructional theory and research.* Alexandria, VA: Association for Supervision and Curriculum Development.

Joyce, B. R. & Weil, M. (1996). *Models of Teaching.* Fifth Edition. Boston: Allyn and Bacon.

Kestenberg, J. (1995). *Sexuality, body movement and the rhythms of development.* Norvale, NJ: Jason Aronson, Inc.

Kalish, B. (1974). Body movement for autistic children. *ADTA Combined Proceedings for the 3rd and 4th Annual Conference* (pp. 49–59). Columbia, MD: American Dance Therapy Association.

Kernberg, O. (1976) *Object relations: Theory and clinical psychoanalysis.* New York: Jason Aronson.

Kohut, H. (1971). *Analysis of the self.* New York: International Universities Press.

Kohut, H. (1977). *Restoration of the self.* New York: International Universities Press.

Koren, B.-S. (1994). A concept of "body knowledge" and an evolving model of "movement experience": Implications and applications for curriculum and teacher education. *American Journal of Dance Therapy, 16*(1), 21–48.

Kroll, J. (1997). Psychotherapy of borderline patients. In M. Rosenbluth, (Ed.) (1997). *Treating difficult personality disorders* (pp. 81–106). San Francisco: Jossey-Bass Inc., Publisher.

Krueger, D. W. & Schofield, E. (1986). Dance/movement therapy of eating disordered patients: A model. *The Arts in Psychotherapy, 13,* 323–331.

Kurtz, R. (1990). *Body-centered psychotherapy,* Mendocino, CA: LifeRhythm.

Laban, R. (1971). *Mastery of movement.* London: The Whitefriars Press Ltd.

Lamb, W. (1965). *Posture and gesture: An introduction to the study of physical behaviour.* London: Gerald Duckworth & Co., Ltd.

Lambert, M. J., & Bergin, A. E. (1994). The effectiveness of psychotherapy. In Bergin, A. E. and Garfield, S. L. (Eds.). *Handbook of Psychotherapy and Behavior Change.* 4th Edition. (pp. 143–189). New York: John Wiley and Sons, Inc.

Lasseter, J., Privette, G., Brown, C. C., and Duer, J. (1989). Dance as treatment approach with a multidisabled child: Implications for school counseling. *The School Counselor, 36,* 310–315.

Lefco, H. (1974). *Dance/movement therapy: Narrative case histories of therapy sessions of with six patients.* Chicago: Nelson Hall.

Leventhal, F. & Chang, M. (1991). Dance/movement therapy with battered women: A paradigm of action. *American Journal of DanceTherapy, 13*(2), 131–145.

Levy, F. J. (1988). *Dance/movement therapy: A healing art.* Reston, VA: National Dance Association and American Alliance for Health, Physical Education, Recreation, and Dance.

Lewis, P. (1984). *Theoretical approaches in dance-movement therapy.* Volume II. Dubuque, Iowa: Kendall Hunt Publishers.

Lewis, P. (1986). *Theoretical approaches in dance-movement therapy.* Volume I. Dubuque, Iowa: Kendall Hunt Publishers.

Lewis, P. (1996). Depth psychotherapy in dance/movement therapy. *American Journal of DanceTherapy 18*(2), 95–114.

Liebowitz, G. (1992). Individual dance movement therapy in an inpatient psychiatric setting. In H. Payne, (Ed.). *Dance movement therapy: Theory and practice.* New York and London: Routledge.

Lindner, E. C. (1982). Dance as a therapeutic intervention for the elderly. *Educational gerontology 8,* 167–174.

Links, P. S., Steiner, M., & Offord, D. R., et al. (1988). Characteristics of borderline personality disorder: A Canadian study. *Canadian Journal of Psychiatry, 33,* 336–340.

Lowen, A. (1967). *Betrayal of the body,* New York: Macmillan.

Macdonald, B. J. (Ed.). (1995). *Theory as a prayerful act.* New York: Peter Lang.

Mahler, M. S. (1968). *On human symbiosis and the vicissitudes of individuation.* New York: International Universities Press.

Mahler, M. S., Pine, F., & Bergmann, A. (1975). *The psychological birth of the human infant.* London: Hutchinson.

Mason, K. C. (Eds.). (1974). *Dance/movement therapy.* Washington, DC: American Alliance for Health, Physical Education, and Recreation.

Masterson, J. (1981). *The narcissistic and borderline disorders.* New York: Brunner/Mazel.

Metronews. (1973). *Chicago-Reed mental health center newsletter, 5*(14), 1–4. February 15, 1973.

Meyer, S. (1985). Women and conflict in dance therapy. *Women and Therapy, 4* (1), 3–16.

Milliken, R. (1990). Dance/movement therapy with the substance abuser. *The Arts in Psychotherapy, 17,* 309–317.

Minuchin, S., Rosman, B. L., & Baker, L. (1978). *Psychosomatic families: Anorexia nervosa in context.* Cambridge, MA: Harvard University Press.

Nigg, J. T., Silk, K. R., Westen, D., et al. (1991). Object representations in the early memories of sexually abused borderline patients. *American Journal of Psychiatry, 148,* 846–896.

North, M. (1995). Marian Chace Annual Lecture: Catch the Pattern. *American Journal of DanceTherapy, 17*(1), 5–14.

Ogata, S. N., Silk, K. R., & Goodrich, S. (1990). The childhood experience of the borderline patient. In *Family Environment and Borderline Personality Disorder.* (Ed. P. Links). Washington, DC: American Psychiatric Press.

Ornstein, A. C. & Hunkins, F. P. (1998). *Curriculum: Foundations, principles, and issues* (3rd ed.), Boston, MA; Allyn and Bacon.

Partelli, L. (1995). Aesthetic listening: Contributions of dance/movement therapy to the psychic understanding of motor stereotypes and distortions in autism and psychosis in childhood and adolescence. *The Arts in Psychotherapy, 22,* 241–247.

Payne, H. (Ed.). (1992). *Dance/movement therapy: Past and present.* London, New York, Tavistock/Routledge.

Payne, H. (1988). The use of dance/movement therapy with troubled youth. (pp. 68–97). In C. E. Schaefer (Ed.). *Innovative Interventions in Child and Adolescent Therapy.* New York: Wiley

Perlmutter, M. A. (1992). The dance of addiction. *American Journal of DanceTherapy, 14*(1), 41–48.

Perry, J. (1994). Cloning Socrates. *Performance and instruction. 33,* 10–11.

Perry, S. Cooper, A. M., & Michels, R. (1987). Psychodynamic formulation: Its purpose, structure, and clinical application. *American Journal of Psychiatry, 144*(5), 543–550.

Rauskin, A. (1990). A dance/movement therapy model of incorporating movement education with emotionally disturbed children. *The Arts in Psychotherapy, 17,* 55–67.

Reiland, J. D. (1990). A preliminary study of dance/movement therapy with field-dependent alcoholic women. *The Arts in Psychotherapy, 17,* 349–354.

Richey, R. (1992). *Designing instruction for the adult learner.* London: Kogan Page Ltd.

Ritter, M. & Low, K, G. (1996). Effects of Dance/movement therapy: A meta-analysis. *The Arts in Psychotherapy, 23*(3), 249–260.

Romero, E. F., Hurwitz, A., & Carranza, V. (1983). Dance therapy on a therapeutic community for schizophrenic patients. *The Arts in Psychotherapy, 10,* 85–92.

Rosenbluth, M. (1997). *Treating difficult personality disorders.* San Francisco, CA: Jossey-Bass Publishers.

Rosenthal, R. (1984). Meta-analytic procedures for social research.

Beverly Hills, CA: Sage.

Rossberg-Gempton, I., & Poole, G. D. (1992). The relationship between body movement and affect: From historical and current perspectives. *The Arts in Psychotherapy, 19,* 39–46.

Samberg, S. (1988). Dance therapy groups for the elderly. In B. W. Maclennan, S. Saul, M. B. Weiner (Eds.), with J. E. Blum, M. Linden, & J. Skigen (1988). *Group psychotherapies for the elderly.* (pp. 233–243). Madison: International Universities Press, Inc.

Sandel, S. L. (1978). Movement therapy with geriatric patients in a convalescent home. *Hospital and community psychiatry, 29*(11), 738–741.

Sandel, S. L., Chaiklin, S., & Lohn, A. (Eds.). (1993). *Foundations of dance/movement therapy: The life and work of Marian Chace.* Columbia, MD: Marian Chace Memorial Fund of the American Dance Therapy Association.

Satir, V. & Baldwin, M. (1983). *Satir step by step.* Palo Alto, CA: Science and Behavior Books, Inc.

Saul, S. (1988). The arts as psychotherapeutic modalities with groups of older people. In B. W. Maclennan, S. Saul, M. B. Weiner (Eds.), with J. E. Blum, M. Linden, & J. Skigen (1988). *Group psychotherapies for the elderly.* (pp. 211–221). Madison: International Universities Press, Inc.

Schlesginer, H. J, Mumford, E., & Glass, G. V. (1978). *A critical review and indexed bibliography of the literature to 1978 on the effects of psychotherapy on medical utilization.* Denver: University of Colorado Medical Center.

Schilder, P. (1925). *The image and appearance of the human body.* England: Routledge & Kegan Paul.

Schilder, P. (1950). *The image and appearance of the human body.* New York: International Universities Press.

Schoop, T. (1974). *Won't you join the dance? A dancer's essay into the treatment of psychosis.* Palo Alto, CA: Mayfield Publishing Company.

Schoop, T. and Michell, P. (1986). Reflections and projections: The Schoop approach to dance therapy. In P. Lewis. (1986). *Theoretical approaches in dance-movement therapy.* Volume I. Dubuque, Iowa: Kendall Hunt Publishers.

Schulman, L. S. (1999). Knowledge and teaching: Foundations of the new reform. In A. C. Ornstein & L. S. Behar-Horenstein, (Eds.). *Contemporary issues in curriculum.* (pp. 103–121). Needham Heights, MA: Allyn & Bacon.

Schwarz, E. D., & Perry, B. D. (1994). The post-traumatic response in children and adolescents. *Psychiatric clinics of North America, 17*(2), 311–326.

Schur, M. (1955). Comments on the metapsychology of somatization. *The Psychoanalytic study of the child, 10*, 119–164. New York: International Universities Press.

Seligman, M. P. (1995). The effectiveness of psychotherapy: The Consumer Reports study. *American Psychologist, 50*(12), 965–974.

Shennum, W. A. (1987). Expressive activity therapy in residential treatment: Effects on children's behavior in the treatment milieu. *Child & Youth Quarterly, 16*(2), 81–90.

Siegel, E. V. (1988). *Dance/movement therapy: Mirror of ourselves.* New York: Human Science Press.

Siegel, E. V. (1973). Movement therapy as a psychotherapeutic tool. *Journal of the American Psychoanalytic Association, 21*(2), 333–343.

Slavin, R. E. (1986). An alternative to meta-analysis and traditional reviews. *Educational Researcher 15*(9), 5–11.

Snow, R. E. (1973). Theory construction for research on teaching. In R. M. Travers (Ed.), *Second handbook of research on teaching.* Chicago: Rand McNally.

Spradley, J. P. (1980). Participant observation. New York: Holt.

Stanton, K. (1991). Dance/movement therapy: An introduction. *British Journal of Occupational Therapy, 54*(3), 108–110.

Sullivan, H. S. (1953). *The interpersonal theory of psychiatry.* New York: Norton.

Sullivan, H. S. (1964). *The fusion of psychiatry and social science.* New York: Norton.

Tarleton, D. (1992). *Dimensions of learning: A model for enhancing student thinking and learning.* Washington, DC: (ERIC Document ED361 326)

Thomson, D. (1997). Dance/movement therapy with the dual-diagnosed: A vehicle to the self in the service of recovery. *American Journal of Dance Therapy, 19*(1), 63–79.

Young, T. A. (1986). *Trudi Schoop: From dance mime to dance/movement therapy.* M.A. Thesis, Texas Women's University.

Weiner, J. (1985). Creative movement with the learning disabled child. *Journal of reading, writing, and learning disabilities international, 1*(3), 34–44.

Westbrook, B. K., & McKibben, H. (1989). Dance/movement therapy with groups of outpatients with Parkinson's disease. *American Journal of Dance Therapy, 11*(1), 27–38.

Westmeyer, P. (1988). *Effective teaching in adult and higher education.* Springfield, IL: Charles C. Thomas Publisher.

Whitehouse, M. S. (1986). C. G. Jung and dance therapy: Two major principles. In P. Lewis. *Theoretical approaches in dance-movement therapy.* Volume I. (pp. 61–85). Dubuque, Iowa: Kendall Hunt Publishers.

Winnicott, D. (1965). The maturational process and pathological narcissism. London: Hogarth Press.

Wise, S. K. (1981). Integrating the use of music in movement therapy for patients with spinal cord injuries. *American Journal of Dance Therapy, 4*(1), 42–51.

Witkin, H. A., Moore, C. A., Goodenough, D. R., & Cox, P. W. (1977). Field dependent and independent cognitive styles and their educational implications. *Review of Educational Research, 47*(1) 1–64.

Wolberg, A. (1982). *Psychoanalytic and psychotherapy of the borderline patient.* (p. 226). New York: Thieme-Stratton.

Yalom, I. D. (1975). *The theory and practice of group psychotherapy.* New York: Basic Books.

Zanarini, M., Gunderson, J. G. & Frankenburg, F. R., et al. (1989). Childhood experiences of borderline patients. *Comprehensive Psychiatry, 30,* 18–25.

Proclamation from the Mayor of Chicago

OFFICE OF THE MAYOR
CITY OF CHICAGO

HAROLD WASHINGTON
MAYOR

PROCLAMATION

WHEREAS, the 21st Annual Conference "Coming of Age," of the American Dance Therapy Association will be held Wednesday, November 5 through Sunday, November 9, at the Holiday Inn Mat Plaza; and

WHEREAS, dance/movement therapists are employed in a wide range of facilities, work with diverse populations, and address the needs of a broad spectrum of specific disorders and disabilities; and

WHEREAS, Jane Ganet-Sigel, a 21 year pioneer in Dance Therapy, founder and director of the Columbia College Dance Therapy Graduate Program, therapist in private practice and the first Dance Therapist in the Chicagoland and midwestern areas, is being honored at this Conference; and

WHEREAS, Mrs. Ganet-Sigel's tenacity and loyalty to both her profession and hometown has resulted in Dance Therapy's flourishing here as a respected and valuable tool for treating individuals with psychological disorders:

NOW, THEREFORE, I, Harold Washington, Mayor of the City of Chicago, do hereby proclaim November 5–9, 1986 to be "COMING OF AGE" — JANE GANET-SIGEL DAY IN CHICAGO in recognition of the 21st Annual Conference "Coming of Age" and for the many contributions of Chicagoans and midwestern Dance Therapists, such as Jane Ganet-Sigel, for devotion to development and growth in this field.

Dated this 27th day of October, 1986

[signed "Harold Washington"]
Mayor

Index

A

abstract cognition, 149
active learners, 93
active learning, 107
addiction, 175
Adler, J., 176
ADTA, ix, xii, xv, 2, 10, 39, 40, 49, 201
adult learners, 84, 86, 87
aggression, 111, 144
Allen, J., 184
alternative treatment modalities, xvi
altruism, 27, 55, 68
Alzheimer's disease, xi
Anderson, B., 144
anorexia nervosa, 6, 134, 153, 154, 155
association of registered dance/movement therapist (ADTR), 38
attention to the interactional aspect, 18, 19
attunement, 143
authentic movement, 20
autism, 40
autonomy, 12, 137, 157

B

Baker, L., 154, 155, 164
Baldwin, M., 37
Balint, M., 16
Barnes, C., 87
Barnett, B., 85, 86
Bartenieff, I., 168
basic trust, 12, 136
Baumann, E. H., 40

Beaudry, J. S., 81
Behar-Horenstein, L. S., ix, 71, 141, 187
behavioral family of models, 76
Berelowitz, M., 142, 144
Bergin, A. E., 171
Bergmann, A., 144
Berrol, C., 176
Blanck, G., 5, 142, 143
Blanck, R., 5, 142, 143
Blume, E., 155
body action, 7, 13, 14, 138
body image, 11, 13, 27
body movement, xi
Boerckel, D., 87
Bohlin, R. M., 86, 87
borderline personality disorder, 134, 141, 142, 144
Borg, W. R., 170, 171
Braff, D., 176, 177
Brown, A. K., ix
Brown, C. C., 171
Brown, G. R., 144
Bruch, H., 163
Bryne, C. P., 144
bulimia, 164

C

Caffarella, R., 85, 86
Calhoun, E., 74, 75, 76, 77
Canner, N. G., 180
Cao, L., 53, 179
capacity for intervention, 9
career development, 37
Carranza, V., 168, 176, 177

About the Authors

Linda S. Behar-Horenstein is an associate professor in the Department of Educational Leadership at the University of Florida. She has a Ph.D. in Curriculum and Instruction and an M.A. in Guidance and Counseling. Dr. Behar-Horenstein has published over 25 articles and several book chapters on curriculum theory and practice in schools and higher education, and effective curriculum strategies in teaching and leadership.

She is the author of *The Knowledge Base of Curriculum: An Empirical Analysis,* co-editor of *Paradigm Debates in Curriculum and Supervision: Modern and Postmodern Perspectives* (forthcoming), and co-editor of *Contemporary Issues in Curriculum.* She is also a member of the Professors of Curriculum. She is married to Ben Horenstein and has a daughter, Rachel, and a son, Max who was created and delivered while this book was being written.

Jane Ganet-Sigel is a registered dance movement therapist and one of the 73 founding members of the American Dance/Movement Therapy Association. She is the founder and former chairperson of the graduate program in Dance/Movement Therapy at Columbia College in Chicago. Ganet-Sigel has been a supervisor, teacher, trainer, and private practice therapist. She has conducted workshops through the USA, and in China, Argentina, and Mexico. She is formerly the Director of the Creative Workshop for dance and drama. Ganet-Sigel has worked in and been a consultant to various hospitals, institutions, mental health agencies, and schools, for a variety of patient populations. She is married to Melvin Sigel and has four children, four step-children, twenty-one grandchildren, and two great-grandchildren.